REAL FITNESS!

"Make no mistake about it, Rochelle Rice is the real thing. And the program she's offering here is no less real—the active life you've been putting off, or possibly never thought you could have can be yours. Now. Not after you lose weight. Now."

—Amy, 33, editor

◆

"A year and a half ago, I began the program in REAL FITNESS FOR REAL WOMEN, and from the very first day I began to feel more comfortable with myself. I now work out to get fit—not to lose weight, but to get fit and to move. I was taking medication for high blood pressure. Now I regulate my condition through diet and exercise. I no longer need medication."

—Cynthia, 32, preschool and kindergarten teacher

◆

"I used to join gyms where I'd last a week and then quit. This time, I can't imagine quitting. I feel so much better. I like the fact that I can move and exercise without stopping in the middle because I feel like I am going to collapse. I used to dread the prospect of working out. Now my workout is the high point of my week."

—Leslie, 30, children's therapist

◆

"Working out helped me get back my physical and emotional strength. It was an incredibly empowering experience. It's a lot easier for me to make better food choices as well. I haven't been dieting, I've just become more aware of what I'm eating. And at the end of my workouts, instead of feeling completely exhausted, I feel elated."

—Kathleen, 36, legal secretary

◆

"I tried Optifast, I joined Weight Watchers many times, and earlier in my life I tried diet drugs and amphetamines. The weight never stayed off. . . . Now I have a different attitude about myself and my body. . . . I'm beginning to be aware of my connection to my muscles and my body, as well as to my spirit. I have more stamina, mental clarity, and energy. I feel more alive!"

—Barbara, 56, nurse practitioner

REAL FITNESS FOR REAL WOMEN

A UNIQUE WORKOUT PROGRAM FOR THE PLUS-SIZE WOMAN

Rochelle Rice

WARNER BOOKS

A Time Warner Company

Neither this nor any other exercise program should be followed without first consulting a health care professional. If you have any special conditions requiring attention, you should consult with your health care professional regularly regarding possible modification of the program contained in this book.

Warner Books, Inc., 1271 Avenue of the Americas, New York, NY 10020
Visit our Web site at www.twbookmark.com

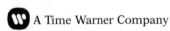 A Time Warner Company

Printed in the United States of America
First Printing: February 2001
10 9 8 7 6 5 4 3 2

Library of Congress Cataloging-in-Publication Data
Rice, Rochelle.
    Real fitness for real women : a unique workout program for the plus size woman / by
    Rochelle Rice with Kathy Silburger.
        p. cm.
    Includes index
    ISBN 0-446-67621-7
    1. Exercise for women. 2. Physical fitness for women. 3. Women—Health and hygiene.
    I. Silburger, Kathy. II. Title.

RA781 .R52 2001
613.7'045—dc21

                                                                                        00-042344

Book design and text composition by Ellen Gleeson
Cover design by Elaine Groh
Photographs by Ira Fox

Dedicated to my grandmother
Eleanor C. Hill,
whose passion and dedication to the joy of movement
forever inspires me.

ACKNOWLEDGMENTS

This project is the culmination of seven years of work with women of size. The project would not have been possible without the help of my family, friends, and, most importantly, my clients.

I would like to express my gratitude to Tanya McKinnon at Mary Evans, Inc., for her high level of professionalism, willingness to take a chance in life, and her unconditional belief in the need for this book. Thank you to Kathy Silburger for her writing expertise—she thanks Dr. J. My sincere thanks to Diana Baroni at Warner Books for embracing this fitness concept for women.

I am grateful to Laura Geller for the make-overs provided for the models and to Laura at Plus Woman for providing the fitness attire. Thank you to Ira Fox for his extraordinary photography and sensitivity. My heartfelt thanks to the book models—Kathleen Fitzmaurice, Anita Franklin, and Marie LeClaire, as well as the women who shared their stories of inspiration . . . Anita, Barbara, Cynthia, Denyse, Kathleen, Leslie, Pat, and Sandy. Your courage and willingness to share your personal stories will inspire other women to lead an active lifestyle.

My thanks to those who were instrumental in inspiring my fitness career—Margaret Prindle for introducing me to the world of fitness, Vincent Cutro for locating my first fitness studio in Greenwich Village, and Dr. Mary McBride for encouraging me to research this work for my master's thesis project at New York University.

I wish to thank my movement mentors, the women who influenced this program: Lynn Simonson for her extraordinary ability to teach dance; Irene Dowd for her anatomical wisdom; and Rebecca Deitzel for her editing and uncanny connection of muscles to movement! I acknowledge Pat Lyons and Debby Burgard, Ph.D., authors of *Great Shape*, as well as the women before me who pioneered the reality of fat and fit.

My deepest respect and gratitude to the women I have had the opportunity to work with. Your trust and willingness to communicate will help champion a day when women will no longer be oppressed by the diet and fitness industry.

With love to my family and friends who have surrounded me with faith and support: to my parents who always made me believe I could be whatever I wanted, to Mom and Dad Fernandez and Steven Fernandez for their unconditional love and support, to Joan Canavan for her mentoring and belief in our generations of powerful women. With love to Alicia Clanton whose smile lights my heart; and to Tina Collin for her friendship, inspiration, and love of life. To Danna Homburger, Heather McDonald, and Rhonda Alexis St. John—thank you for being my beautiful core of strength and sanity. To Howard Teich—thank you for seeing all that I was capable of at such a pivotal point in my life. To the NAAFA Board of Directors, thank you for electing this ally. To Annette Vallano, for her beautiful friendship, wisdom, and support. And to Dr. Agnes Wilkie and Dr. Scott Rogge for the safe space where I could write this book.

My thanks to God and the Divine light which shines within all of us—how grateful I am to have found my flow in life . . . an incredibly rich and rewarding journey . . . powerful beyond my wildest expectations.

CONTENTS

INTRODUCTION

Agnes M. Wilkie, M.D.

I am a physician who specializes in psychiatry. I am also a woman of size. You may be asking yourself: Why should I read yet another book about exercise and fitness? Why should I bother with another exercise program? What's so different about this one?

While the health, fitness, and weight loss industries would have you believe that being thin is the only way to be healthy and fit, this groundbreaking fitness program designed by Rochelle Rice will prove otherwise. *Real Fitness for Real Women* will show you that you can improve your health, fitness, and energy no matter what your size, weight, or waistline may be.

If you're anything like me, you've probably read many books, started more than a few exercise programs, and joined a gym or two in an effort to begin a regular routine of exercise. Your doctor may even have told you to exercise and diet to improve your health and reduce your risk factors for certain diseases.

As a society, we tend to be very goal-directed. We do things to get results, not to enjoy the process. This is no less true of our fitness programs. We exercise to lose weight and look better.

Until my work with Rochelle, I shared this belief that the sole purpose of exercise was to lose weight and inches. I would embark upon a new fitness program at a new gym whenever my clothes felt too snug, or there was a special event at which I wanted to look my best. I viewed the exercises as sheer drudgery, as the painful price I had to pay for the ever-elusive goal of thinness.

Rochelle's program changed all that. And in doing so, it has literally changed my life. What makes Rochelle's program different? This innovative program focuses on exercise and movement rather than diet as a means of attaining fitness. The exercises are specifically designed for the large-sized person. The program also addresses the psychological concerns that these individuals may have about exercise and their bodies.

Rochelle's program not only makes sense, but also is scientifically sound. Medical research has amply demonstrated that being fit confers a broad range of physiological benefits, including:

✦ Decreasing the risk of osteoarthritis
✦ Decreasing the risk of osteoporosis
✦ Enhancing immune function
✦ Increasing oxygen consumption
✦ Improving balance and coordination, thereby reducing the risk of injuries due to falls
✦ Improving blood circulation
✦ Improving sleep
✦ Lowering blood pressure
✦ Lowering the risk of heart disease and stroke
✦ Preventing the development of gallstones
✦ Reducing blood glucose levels and increasing the body's receptivity to insulin to reduce the risk of diabetes

The goal of *Real Fitness for Real Women* is to get you moving so you can begin to experience all of the medical benefits just described. But they can only be attained with a carefully designed program that attends to the unique physique of the plus-size woman. A "one routine fits all sizes" approach just won't do. In fact, such a regimen can be downright dangerous, especially for women of size beginning an exercise program. Too often secondary injuries such as shin splints, calf strains, low back discomfort and knee problems set them back physically and psychologically right at the start. Rochelle's program is carefully designed and paced to help each client develop the strength and flexibility she needs to avoid such early setbacks.

Exercise has many psychological benefits as well. Movement is useful as an outlet for emotion. It has also been shown to:

✦ Decrease anxiety
✦ Decrease depression
✦ Decrease the effects of stress

Exercise also affects many brain chemicals, called neurotransmitters, which have a role in regulating mood. These include serotonin, dopamine, norepinephrine, and endorphins. These are the same chemicals that are impacted by the antidepressant and anti-anxiety medications used to help treat mood disorders.

As a psychiatrist, I take a particular interest in how Rochelle's program might affect one's moods. The link between exercise and mood is not as simple and straightforward as it might seem at first.

When people get depressed they tend to abandon their exercise routines. When the depression starts to lift they return to exercise. It appears that depression represents a loss of psychic and physical energy. What ensues is a need for the human organism to conserve energy. Unfortunately, when people abandon their physical activities it tends to have a negative impact on their energy as well as their self-esteem. This adds to their depressed mood, which perpetuates the negative cycle of depression.

Rochelle Rice developed the program in *Real Fitness for Real Women* to increase overall psychological as well as physical health. It combats these negative cycles because it attends to the special psychological needs of plus-size women. It adopts a supportive, positive, graduated approach that recognizes the importance of safety and success for women who may have come away from other programs feeling embarrassed, incompetent, or even injured. Meditations and other techniques incorporated into the program further build feelings of psychological strength and resiliency, as well as confidence and self-esteem.

Rochelle's program offers other psychological benefits. Unlike other programs, you will find the emphasis placed on exercise for the purpose of feeling good just for its own sake; feeling pleasure in movement; movement as an outlet for emotion; or as a way to feel stronger in your body. This latter perspective of movement in particular is what makes Rochelle's program so bold. She's challenging us to move so that we can enjoy our bodies, our lives, and ourselves more. She welcomes us to improve the quality of our lives through movement. She takes a more practical approach to fitness and relates it to our ordinary daily activities so that we will feel stronger when we climb steps, lift grocery bags, pick up children, and have the energy to stay out late dancing.

This program challenges the traditional fitness and medical industries to redefine what it means to be fit. Her approach emphasizes the many health-giving physical and psychological benefits of exercise, regardless of the size or weight of the participant. This is not to say that weight and size are irrelevant to one's health status. What it means is that an overemphasis on weight loss as the goal of exercise leads many women to become discouraged. As a result, they may not initiate or maintain any exercise regimen at all, or may exercise unsafely and incur injuries.

Real Fitness for Real Women offers women a refreshingly different focus, an entirely new exercise experience. After all, what is clear is that some exercise is better than none, as long as it is performed in an informed and safe manner. And this is what Rochelle Rice gives us in this innovative, groundbreaking, and evolving program which she has researched and designed for plus-size women.

As a psychiatrist, my life's work has been devoted to helping people deal with their difficulties in life. Rochelle's program has been a powerful therapeutic tool that has helped me change my life. I have embraced exercise as a means to greater strength, flexibility, and aerobic stamina. I am more focused, more disciplined, and more self-directed. I have more energy, and feel more powerful. I am stronger and more resilient physically and emotionally. I have greater self-confidence. As a result of this personal growth, I have been able to make important changes in my professional and personal lives, which have brought me greater happiness and fulfillment. I invite you to learn about how *Real Fitness for Real Women* can help you change your life and achieve your goals by empowering you through movement.

PROLOGUE

For most of my life, I was afraid of movement. If friends called to make plans, I'd make a quick mental calculation—if it involved walking a great distance or any significant physical exertion, I declined. Extremely overweight, I knew I would never be able to keep up, and didn't want to call attention to myself. So I sat out, shut myself in, and waited to get thin, allowing myself to believe I was merely the sum of my flesh. The same flesh, meanwhile, frightened, isolated, condemned, and, in some strange way, protected me.

In 1989, twenty-two years old and just out of college, I lost more than 60 pounds on a liquid diet. As part of that program I began to exercise, and for the first time in my life, really move. I had never felt better, and of course attributed that to the weight loss. When the pounds inevitably crept back on, I stopped exercising, as if the "right" to fitness was a luxury only afforded to thin women.

And so it went for years, until I began to worry about my health. Even though my blood pressure, cholesterol, and other vitals were fine, I was always lethargic and depressed. I just didn't feel well. One day I became sick and tired of being sick and tired, and I vowed to get strong.

This time though, I wanted a kinder, gentler path. The pain of gaining back all I'd lost on the liquid diet proved to me that extreme methods didn't work. Much less obsessive than others, I began to notice how consumed my friends and co-workers were with their own quests for thinness. No matter their shape or size, every woman I encountered had her own issues around food and body image. I'm talking about women from a variety of backgrounds and ethnicities—strong, intelligent, highly educated, otherwise well-adjusted women—all spouting the same nonsense: We're "good" if we eat a salad (dressing on the side, of course), "bad" if we indulge in (oh horrors!) ice cream. We're "good" if we work out on the treadmill for one hour, "bad" if we exercise for less than 20 minutes.

Slowly, oh so slowly, I began to block out this nonsense and simply pay attention to when and where my body felt the best. If my legs were sore, I stretched them. If my stomach hurt from eating junk food, I refrained. I began to rely on my own two feet for transportation around the city, enjoying the experience of being among the living, of feeling alive. I was a tender seedling at that point, but I knew it felt right, and for once I followed my instincts.

When I saw an ad for In Fitness & In Health, Rochelle's fitness studio designed for plus-size women, in a local newspaper, I was skeptical. Yet another "program"? Another institutional attempt at fitness? I just didn't want to "fail" again. You went to the gym when you were already fit, to maintain your fitness. I'd been to gyms before. It felt as though everyone was staring at me thinking, "I better keep working out . . . I don't want to end up like her!"—precisely the mentality that kept me, for years, in self-induced solitary confinement.

When I walked into Rochelle's studio for the first time, she greeted me with a warm, open smile. But as warm as Rochelle was, the only thing I could think was, "How could anyone that thin and that perky understand me? What could she possibly know about a body like mine? And why would she even want to?"

The rest of our meeting can best be described by what Rochelle didn't do:

✦ Give me the once-over or the tsk-tsk that plus-size women face every day
✦ Pull out the (dreaded) measuring tape
✦ Promise that I'd be thin "in no time," or that I'd emerge a "whole new me"
✦ Judge, disapprove, or condescend; and, drum roll please . . .
✦ She never asked about my weight—not even a hint, it just was not an issue

I've been working out at In Fitness & In Health for five years now. And I'm a much stronger, healthier, and happier person for it. Since the workouts we do at In Fitness & In Health (and the ones in *Real Fitness for Real Women*) are specifically designed for the plus-size body (and mind), they will help you feel challenged but not defeated. Because you feel positive about yourself, you'll stick with it. Rochelle is a unique individual, and the program she has designed and that she shares in *Real Fitness for Real Women* is truly innovative and inspiring. Through the program, plus-size women will be able to move, breathe, and sweat without feeling self-conscious or pushed too hard—you will feel alive, empowered, and strong. That's what it has done for me. As a plus-size woman, I know how rare it is to walk into a room and not feel as though I have to carve out a safe corner for myself. I know how refreshing it is to not be obsessed with what people think of the size of my hips. Thanks to Rochelle's infectious open-heart and open-mind attitude and her program, I feel better about myself. I now am able to go out and leave my self-criticisms at home.

Make no mistake about it, Rochelle Rice is the real thing. And the program she's offering here is no less real—the active life you've been putting off, or possibly never thought you could have, can be yours. Now. Not after you lose weight. Now.

I have reconnected with the body I'd been avoiding for years. Even though it doesn't have the exact shape and form I'd like, it's thriving. Suddenly I'm moving unencumbered, more efficiently, and not expending unnecessary energy just to get started. Things are easier!

So thank you, Rochelle, for keeping me positive, inspired, and in a perpetual state of perspiration and engaged abdominals. Without further ado, I introduce you to Rochelle Rice—teacher and student, trainer and friend—and the amazing, revolutionary program in *Real Fitness for Real Women*.

—Amy Eiges
five-year student of
Rochelle Rice and her program

REAL
FITNESS FOR
REAL
WOMEN

CHAPTER ONE

MY STORY

*"Our deepest fear is not that we are inadequate. Our deepest fear is that
we are powerful beyond measure. It is our light, not our darkness,
that most frightens us."
We ask ourselves, Who am I to be brilliant, gorgeous, talented, fabulous?
Actually, who are you not to be?
You are a child of God. Your playing small doesn't serve the world.
There's nothing enlightened about shrinking so that other people
won't feel insecure around you. We are all meant to shine, as children do.
We were born to make manifest the glory of God that is within us.
It's not just in some of us; it's in everyone.
And as we let our own light shine, we unconsciously give other people permission
to do the same. As we're liberated from our own fear,
our presence automatically liberates others.*

—Marianne Williamson

I grew up in front of the mirror. I was a dancer from the age of three, and with
each passing year I watched myself more and more critically, scrutinizing my
young form for imperfections. As my body began to develop in adolescence into
a real woman's body, I felt completely alienated by the changes of maturation:
I hated my widening hips, my developing breasts, the curves that seemed to
have softened my form almost overnight. I cried at the onset of my menstrual
cycle. Although I was developing a normal, real, womanly body, when I looked
in the mirror all I could see was deformity, in the form of fat. My body, it
seemed, was monstrous, a betrayal.

Food became my enemy. By the time I was in college, I had become obsessive about counting calories and exercising. I felt I had to dance off every single calorie I consumed. I spent hours in the dance studio, practicing stretches and combinations, all the while thinking, "Just five more pounds . . . then I'll be okay." Day after day I would vow to go on stringent diets in order to purify my body of what I thought of as the visible evidence of my lack of self-control. But as time went on I was less and less able to adhere to a strict diet. As I placed ever more prohibitions on my food and eating, I began to rebel against these violent and self-punishing strictures, bingeing on all the foods I had deemed off limits. Then, guilty at having gorged on fattening foods, I would purge by forcing myself to throw up, nullifying, I thought, the consequences of my moral lapse.

I used to call it "Praying to the Porcelain God," a spirit so powerful it grabbed me by the throat and choked me until the acidic juices from my stomach burned my mouth, every piece of my latest binge expelled. Tears would wash over me, a combination of relief and self-pity. One summer, at a dance camp, a fellow dancer taught me to use laxatives as an alternative to throwing up. I would binge, then swallow handfuls of these pink tablets in order to offset the size of my meal. The following day, gas pains would rip through my gut like knives. But still I went obediently to dance class, trying to maintain the facade that everything was okay.

Instead of dealing with the emotional issues underlying my self-punishing views of my body, it was easier to hide behind the cruel comfort of food. Secretly, like a princess waiting to be rescued, I kept hoping someone would come along and save me from the emotional dragon banging on my door.

But no one and nothing could save me, and in my self-destructiveness I virtually abandoned myself. I used to call my nightly binges "Smashing and Trashing." I would tear through the kitchen like a drug addict looking for a fix, drinking and eating until I was numb. I would pass out without brushing my teeth or washing my face, having attained peace at last.

Emotionally I had hit rock bottom. The peppermint taste of Tums could no longer quell the acidic churning of my bulimic stomach, nor could any binge soothe the ache of my head and heart. Finally I reached out to a trusted friend for help, and she recommended therapy. I had been looking outside of me, externally, for comfort and safety. Every perceived solution had turned to dust in my hands. Now it was time to turn inward.

In therapy I began to pay attention to the feelings that lay beneath my eating disorder. I realized I had internalized the idea that I could never be *enough*—never thin enough, never smart enough, never pretty enough to be "acceptable." Dance was my one saving grace. Despite the toxic, distorted body image issues, I had found an arena where I could express myself. Movement was the one way for me to release my soul.

Therapy also helped me become aware of the effects of living in a society in which we are bombarded every day with images and messages that say thin equals beauty and health, fat equals ugly and sick. The thinner you are the more love you will receive. I came to understand that this diseased social thinking had affected me and women around me; women like me who were torturing themselves in vain attempts to conform to unhealthy and unrealistic ideals.

In the process of my recovery, I detonated every idea I'd ever had about beauty, desirability, and value—I had to. I wanted a life that was joyful, and not ruled by pain. As my recovery progressed, I began to realize what being female, healthy, and alive really meant. It meant being in tune with my body, not working against it. It meant embracing who I really was. In fact it was through a movement regimen that my recovery took root. I continued to dance and I became a certified fitness trainer with the American Council on Exercise. The more I learned about fitness and understood about my eating disorder, the healthier I got. I wanted to share my new understanding with those who were killing themselves to meet societal pressures concerning their weight. And, most important, those treated worst in our fat-phobic culture: women of size.

I knew the statistics: Nearly half of all American women are overweight. Every year Americans spend over $30 billion on the diet industry, yet every year the number of overweight people increases. If the average woman on the street wears at least a size 12, why weren't any of these women members of the gym I belonged to, or clients in my work as a personal trainer? Where were the real women, and why weren't they represented?

I decided to visit other gyms and health clubs to see if mine was somehow an exception, but it was the same thing again and again. Virtually all gyms and fitness programs totally ignored women of size. It was as if the whole fitness profession had labeled plus-size women as beyond help, or even unworthy of fitness—at least until they lost weight! I believed a unique fitness program to help real women learn how to be fit and healthy, no matter what they weigh, was long overdue.

Many of us know that thinness does not equal physical fitness, but numerous exercise and diet gurus—the people who claim to know the most about health—seem to focus on weight loss at the expense of overall health. No one had created a comprehensive anatomical approach to exercise *specifically* for women of size. I conceived my fitness studio, In Fitness & In Health, and the *Real Fitness for Real Women* program to fill this void—they were created with the needs of real women in mind.

My first step was to study the body mechanics of women of size. I then devised a physiologically sound program for increasing strength, movement, and aerobic capacity. When I saw my individual clients make great strides in a regimen based on my independent research, I decided to get the credentials I needed. I earned a master's degree in individualized study at New York University, allowing me to research and design a program specifically for women of size. The end result? *Real Fitness for Real Women*, which contains the best program for enhancing the physical well-being and quality of life for women of size.

When I started my research, conventional wisdom held that weight loss was a prerequisite of fitness. Women of size had to lose weight first before they could really start getting fit. When I argued that women can achieve fitness at *any* size, that fitness was not about weight but about the body, mind, and spirit, many fitness professionals actually told me I was crazy. But when I offered proof, my fitness colleagues took note. My philosophy is simple: Women don't have to be thin to be fit. Some women may be slender and healthy, but one does not guarantee the other.

I opened my first In Fitness & In Health studio immediately after receiving my degree, and within a year and a half I had opened a second location. I appeared on *Weekend Today in New York* in December 1998. The response was overwhelming. I was inundated with calls from women thanking me for having the courage to articulate what they instinctively knew: The fitness industry discriminates against women of size. These women were relieved to find a fitness program that would regard them as the norm and treat them with respect.

Unfortunately not all women have access to my studios or even the time to schedule regular classes. But although many expensive health clubs and exercise programs would have you believe otherwise, getting fit is something you can do in your own home, right now. In *Real Fitness for Real Women*, I have outlined the same successful program that we teach in my studios. Despite the punishing "no pain no gain" doctrine of our culture, fitness should *not* be intimidating or painful. The women who have followed my program have told me that after just six weeks they have more mobility and stamina and are living fuller, happier, healthier lifestyles.

The program in *Real Fitness for Real Women* consists of a series of exercises tailored to the physiological and psychological needs of plus-size women. The program is designed to help you modify exercises if necessary and correct weaknesses and injuries that may be associated with larger bodies. Since fitness is as much about patterns of thinking as it is about discipline, I offer self-empowerment techniques that will help you develop a healthier, more agile, and more powerful body.

Leading a physically fit life often will result in weight loss, but that is not the primary goal of *Real Fitness for Real Women*. By embarking on my program, you will learn how to:

✦ Achieve your full physical potential
✦ Increase your physical productivity and activities of daily living
✦ Enhance your immune system
✦ Increase your self-esteem
✦ Heal weight-related injuries and discomfort
✦ Enhance your energy, stamina, and quality of life

Instead of taking a pounds-and-inches approach, *Real Fitness for Real Women* takes the focus off dieting and puts it where it belongs: on empowering women through movement. Before you know it, you will have an increased awareness of your body and how it functions, and a sense of your grace and power. You will realize that fitness and beauty can be found in women of any size. This program will change your life!

More than an exercise manual, this book has a much grander theme woven throughout—that of a collective consciousness. As we redefine fitness and health, we begin to restructure the thoughts of all women in terms of shape and size. I often liken it to a pebble thrown in the water, making ripples that widen out through the lake. Each woman who takes an action to change her life affects the lives of women around her. We are in charge of our own destinies; we have the power to strengthen our own self-worth and self-esteem as well as that of others.

Through *Real Fitness for Real Women*, you will regain your strength, increase your quality of life, and enjoy your activities of daily living with a fit and strong body. Remember, you are not a number, nor a size—just real. Your spirit will burst forth, breaking the chains of inactivity. You are not alone—we are here for you. You will not fail. The secret is movement.

CHAPTER TWO

A DIFFERENT APPROACH

*Next to physical survival, the greatest need of a human being
is psychological survival—to be understood, to be affirmed, to be validated,
to be appreciated.*

—Stephen Covey, *The 7 Habits of Highly Effective People*

By now you've probably tried every diet and fitness program out there, only to be disappointed every time they fell short of your needs. You've put down your money for a gym membership, never to return. I am here to tell you the truth about why the diet and fitness world fails plus-size women—not why you fail them.

Like many other plus-size women across America, you recognize that the fitness industry, with its relentless focus on getting thin to be healthy, is not equipped to help you. But I can. My program is accessible and achievable. The exercises are based on an anatomical approach, which lengthens and strengthens the muscles that may be affected by size. *Real Fitness for Real Women* was written specifically for you, the large woman—physically, emotionally, psychologically, and spiritually.

Be assured that my program is different from the rest. I will not tell you to count calories or perform punishing exercises that are uncomfortable or physically impossible. If you follow my program, by the end of just six weeks your body will feel immeasurably better, your spirit will be uplifted, and your fitness level will have improved to such an extent that you will be performing, with ease, tasks and activities you previously thought impossible, such as climbing stairs, being able to walk distances without shortness of breath, or even riding a bicycle.

If you feel like a refugee of the fitness industry, that is, completely alienated by the idea of working out, don't worry—the majority of my clients come to me feeling the same way. Having spent seven years studying the biomechanics of plus-size women, and having worked closely with thousands of women of size, I provide a program that makes sense. The proof is in my many plus-size clients who have been with me for years. There is passion in the eyes of a woman as she awakens to the youthful memories of movement she holds close to her heart. I have watched countless women move from sedentary lifestyles into healthful activity once they have made this connection. The level of mastery that can be achieved is truly extraordinary.

I can make these promises because I have seen it happen time and time again. Thousands of women have come to me as a last resort, after everything else failed, only to find that the program in *Real Fitness for Real Women* is what they've been looking for all along. By embarking on the program, you are part of a sisterhood of women who are fed up with receiving second-class treatment when it comes to fitness and health.

Women of size have never been understood, affirmed, validated, or appreciated by the fitness industry. Until now. How many of you have decided to wait until you've lost weight before you venture into a gym, or maybe you've put your money down for a membership, only never to return? In an ideal world, the gym is a place to get fit, a place without judgment or competition, where one can learn proper physical conditioning and technique. But with its relentless focus on thinness, the typical gym attitude pushes real people further and further away, intimidating them into staying at home.

It takes a tremendous amount of effort to walk into the typical health club as a plus-size woman and face a staff of size 4 "gym cuties" in skintight leotards and a studio of confusing equipment. The walls may be decorated with pictures of women with unrealistically buffed and pumped-up bodies. And because most trainers are small, large women are not given the option of working with real trainers—trainers who are more likely to show, by example, what a plus-size body is capable of achieving.

The very presence of a larger woman seems to make the trainers and other members uncomfortable. Skinny women who have bought into society's beauty myths and are obsessed with losing 5 or 10 pounds may look at you with fear or prejudice.

While the fitness industry would like women to blame themselves for failing to look like Hollywood superstars, I know better. In fact, much of the blame rests on the fitness industry itself. In the gyms, fitness programs have not been properly designed for you—the majority of American women! Many—perhaps most—trainers simply do not understand how to move a woman of size through space. Larger women's bodies may not produce the same speed, biomechanics, and functions as a smaller frame. Therefore a program designed for smaller clients cannot be applied to all body types.

For example, exercises that require a client to get down to and up from the floor may be a hardship. A trainer who understands how the large body moves should offer the plus-size woman a program optimally beneficial to her. However, most trainers simply ask her to do the same series of exercises he or she would teach anyone else. When the woman discovers she cannot do these exercises, she feels she has failed. How can your self-esteem be enhanced through fitness, when the programs out there are set up to make you feel like a failure?

When most trainers begin working with a woman of size, they relentlessly focus on weight loss, ignoring the most important part of her—her spirit. Their goal is to make her thinner, and they neglect the more important goal of overall health and fitness. They're trying to get your body to fit *their program*, rather than devising a program to fit *your body*. These routine disappointments with the very institutions purported to improve your health do little to nurture your spirits. Thus through physiological and psychological neglect, the fitness industry continues to drive larger women further from health.

The medical profession often colludes in this neglect by subscribing to myths about plus-size people, and allowing a focus on weight to eclipse issues of health. Many large, healthy women are told they must lose weight, even when all other indicators such as blood pressure and cholesterol are normal. As a result, many of you put off routine medical checkups because you do not want or need to be chastised about your size.

That was certainly Marie's experience. At approximately 300 pounds, Marie was extremely fit, working out at least three days a week and playing racquetball every weekend. But during an annual checkup her doctor reviewed her statistics three times, shaking his head each time with disbelief that the numbers for her blood pressure, heart rate, and cholesterol were so good. Finally he told her, "Well, you appear to be healthy, but you really should lose some weight."

When new clients come to me, I explain that this alienation has created a disconnection between bodies, minds, and spirits. My goal and passion is to unite them during the six-week program. Slowly, through successive workout sessions, we reawaken the senses of the body as well as create a sense of connectedness physically, emotionally, and spiritually.

For many of you the prospect of embarking on a fitness program and getting in touch with your body is terrifying. The *Real Fitness for Real Women* program is designed to take those hesitations into account. Any woman, at any fitness level, can benefit from this program, from the woman who walks a mile every day to the one who has trouble walking a single city block. This program is not about seeing how hard you can push yourself, or performing punishing routines. It's not about "no pain no gain" or "feel the burn." It's about gently reconnecting you with your body and increasing the number of daily activities you are able to perform. This increased movement will often result in weight loss, but again, that is *not* the ultimate goal of the program—it's an added benefit.

When you hear about my program or first pick up this book, you may initially feel anxious, nervous, or distrustful. This is understandable; the fitness industry is rife with false claims. One videotape promises to magically melt inches; another offers abs of steel. You instinctively recognize these advertising come-ons as empty promises. My approach may be less sensationalized, because I am not hawking a quick fix or promising to change your silhouette overnight. But I can promise this: You will slowly begin to feel success in your ability to move freely. You will stand taller, walk prouder, and feel stronger. As you feel more and more entitled to lead an active lifestyle, your self-esteem will improve. And you will gain a sense of camaraderie with the hundreds of thousands of American women who are slowly changing society's paradigm of what plus-size women are capable of physically achieving.

By freeing yourself from the trap of self-judgment and condemnation based on weight standards, self-esteem takes root. For too long you have judged yourself based on a number on a scale, instead of by a myriad of other qualities such as your interests, your talents, your ability to love. We can now turn our backs on the punishing standards and redefine success on our terms. This is how the journey begins.

Know that you are worthy and entitled to an exercise program that is specifically designed for your body, your spirit. This program is a journey back to *you* filled with self-care and love. For those of you who have never encountered a fitness program that accorded you the respect you deserve, *Real Fitness for Real Women* is the answer. The program commands your respect, dignity, and honor, much like a marriage vow. Keep it close, follow it, use it as a journal. Don't hesitate to underline or to make notes in the margins. Perhaps you can share it with friends and family. It can even be a useful tool for your trainers, who may not understand the biomechanics of women of size.

Remember, movement is liberation. As my client Amy Eiges so succinctly puts it: "With movement comes incredible freedom. It seems the more I move the more other areas of my life become enriched, the more life I breathe into long-dormant goals. And the more fit I become, the easier it is to pick myself up, both literally and figuratively, to move along and work things out."

Movement will transform you, bringing you ever closer to who you are and all that you are meant to be. You don't necessarily have to lose weight to get fit, nor do you have to be in pain all the time. Fitness is not something you experience an hour each week in a classroom. My program teaches you to be aware of how fitness affects your everyday life, every time you play with your kids or climb a flight of stairs or even sit with correct posture in an office chair and breathe deeply. True fitness is not about weighing 130 pounds, or sweating profusely. It is about feeling good, breathing deep, standing tall, walking proud—and empowering yourself through movement!

CHAPTER THREE

GETTING MOTIVATED

Like a muscle, courage is strengthened by use.
—Ruth Gordon

I firmly believe that if we put our minds to something there's absolutely nothing we can't achieve. I have seen this time and again among the women I work with at In Fitness & In Health. When women who have internalized negative societal messages start living healthy, active lifestyles, they almost immediately feel more motivated, energetic, and capable.

The series of techniques upon which the program in *Real Fitness for Real Women* is based are grounded in self-esteem. Self-esteem is the foundation upon which we build our lives, and the primary tool for motivation to change. Just as women of *any* size can suffer from a lack of self-esteem, so too can they possess it. Self-esteem means taking a quiet pride in who you are and in knowing that your identity and worth transcend your body shape. It is self-love and self-care that make you beautiful. And . . . these are what motivate you to get up, honor your body, and get physically fit.

Many of us need a little help in strengthening the "muscles" of self-love and self-esteem; after all, we are works in progress. Like peeling off the papery layers from an onion, improving self-esteem means becoming aware of the layers of self-doubt and criticism we have taken on from the world. In this program we make a commitment to embracing ourselves as we are, to making positive changes in our lives, and to living the most active lives that we can. You may, at times, be challenged by your family and friends if you do not lose significant amounts of weight after beginning this program. However, you may receive accolades of praise for your newfound energy without losing a pound!

Often, a sedentary lifestyle compromises self-esteem because you become disconnected from your body. Like a treasured object sinking slowly into the sea, your awareness of your body falls further and further away from you. You become accustomed to a certain physical numbness, and inactivity becomes the norm.

But that habit of inactivity can be reversed through self-esteem. Self-esteem must be built up like a muscle group—slowly and gently, with love, patience, and respect. Reprogramming a dormant sense of self is a wonderful, motivating process. Certainly you'll have setbacks, but make the commitment to keep moving forward. Surround yourself with people (trainers, family, friends) who understand, validate, and appreciate you, and affirm your efforts to get fit. Read size acceptance literature that supports you in your journey. Connect with other women who have similar goals. You'll discover a renewed sense of well-being and joy.

We never abandon a child who is learning to walk and falls down frequently in the process. Similarly, you must not judge yourself as a failure or abandon yourself in your efforts to get fit. Keep giving yourself positive reinforcement. By following the guidelines of this program you will surely succeed.

Imagine that each of us has a dialogue running inside our heads, quietly broadcasting messages about who and what we are and how we are meant to feel about ourselves or how to be in the world. Learning to access this dialogue can be your most important skill for helping you to improve your life and your health. Like your own internal cheerleading squad, it can lift you up when you need a little extra encouragement, counteract negativity and criticism, and allow you to see yourself as confident and beautiful.

In fact, that dialogue is broadcasting now, even as you read this book. If you could hear the dialogue speaking aloud, what would it say? Perhaps something optimistic: "I hope *Real Fitness for Real Women* works, I'm going to try it." Or you might hear something negative: "You can't do it—you'll never be fit. You've failed before and you'll fail again." It might give voice to your suspicions: "Why should I trust Rochelle? She doesn't know what I'm going through." By accessing this dialogue directly instead of allowing our unconscious to play whatever messages it wishes, we can harness the power within to change our outlook, our actions, and our spiritual, mental, and physical health.

In the past, you may have unconsciously allowed toxic messages from other people to reinforce negative ideas you have about yourself. By internalizing society's view of plus-size women as unacceptable and unhealthy, you have played the negative message over and over again, impairing your efforts to feel good about yourself and take positive actions in your life. The best tool for counteracting poor self-esteem and getting motivated is the use of affirmations and power phrases.

Like a sudden ocean breeze on the hottest day of summer, affirmations and power phrases have the strength to change the climate of our emotions, stripping away negative messages and replacing them with positive ones. By helping us to love ourselves better, they give us immediate and measurable results. Throughout this book, you will notice that I have incorporated some of my favorite power phrases at the start of each chapter. Start using them now, and reap the benefits of this important life tool immediately.

Some people may be put off by the New Age associations they have with affirmations. But there is nothing mysterious in the way they function. You need not believe in anything spiritual or metaphysical in order to utilize the power of affirmations, nor need you believe in God or in any sort of higher power. Affirmations work on your own subconscious, clearing your mind of barriers toward living a fuller, happier life and achieving the results you want. By working on the subconscious level to affect the way you feel about yourself and the world around you, affirmations actually change your thinking patterns, inspiring you to action.

One of my clients who learned to harness the power of affirmations is Randy, who assists a research director at a brokerage firm. Randy had tried to get fit several times, but never found a program she was comfortable with. When she began the *Real Fitness for Real Women* program and started writing affirmations, her commitment to fitness firmly took root. Randy began by placing a blackboard by her bed, and copying her favorite quote: "Let go of the pain of the past, so we can embrace the future with hope," by the writers Kerry Olitzky and Rachel Sabath. Randy began writing other positive messages to herself and placing them in areas where she would be certain to see them: on the bathroom mirror, above the kitchen sink. Spurred on by her affirmations and her fitness routine, Randy lives a more active and healthier life today.

Affirmations are a proven tool of countless successful people. Actors, singers, businesspeople, even world leaders utilize affirmations to help direct themselves toward their goals. Why reinvent the wheel? These positive messages continually remind you that you are perfect exactly as you are and are capable of getting fit. You do not need to lose 100 pounds to feel better or to begin a fitness program. Your body is a precious vehicle that deserves to be taken care of and thanked for carrying you through this world. You care for your body and spirit by surrounding yourself with positive, loving messages and thoughts, and by embracing fitness in your lifestyle.

WRITTEN AFFIRMATIONS

Affirmations may be inspiring quotes by others, words of hope and inspiration that are uplifting and affirming of the human spirit. Or you can make up your own affirmations by writing positive messages to yourself, such as "My body is healthy and strong," or "I give myself permission to move forward in life with ease." Be sure to write these messages in the present, so that you can live them in the moment, rather than envisioning a better future while denying yourself love and acceptance in the present. Reciting or reading these affirmations will clear the way for the positive things you want to occur in your life today.

Copy the affirmations on index cards and put them in places where you are likely to see them—such as the medicine cabinet so you can read them every time you brush your teeth; the bedroom dresser or nightstand; on your mirrors. Use them as bookmarks, or tape them to your kitchen cupboards. Change them if you no longer pay attention to them. You need to constantly stimulate your self-esteem and self-worth, and affirmations are a marvelous tool. The successful people I know can recite these empowering phrases off the top of their heads. Take what successful, strong, self-esteemed people are already doing and apply it to your life—now!

Return to your affirmations and power phrases when you are having a rough day or when you are not inspired. Draw strength from them. They are powerful and will subconsciously continue to reprogram your belief system. When you feel depressed, an affirmation or power phrase can change your mood by reminding you of what you value most, turning despair into reflection and hope.

Share the affirmations with your children. Create the habit so they learn self-esteem and self-worth early in their lives. To give your affirmations added power, try mirroring—or looking at yourself in the mirror as you recite affirmations. While I know that it is difficult for many of us to look in the mirror and recite to ourselves, the results are tremendous. Children are much better at this than adults because they maintain a playful spirit and are natural actors. I think about my eleven-year-old Fresh Air Fund child Alicia, who comes to stay with me in the summer. Every morning and every evening, when she finishes brushing her teeth, we look in the mirror and say, "I am beautiful inside and outside." I pray that as she grows to be a teenager and young adult, the nurturing seeds of self-esteem will blossom throughout adulthood.

HOW TO WRITE YOUR OWN AFFIRMATIONS

Determine the areas in your life or aspects of your self-esteem that you would like to improve. These might include:

✦ A better body image
✦ The confidence to make healthy choices
✦ Increased energy and motivation

Now, close your eyes and picture yourself with that goal met, right this very moment! Picture yourself waking up full of health and vitality, striding down the street with confidence, tackling challenging tasks, and embracing your physical power. Now write down a phrase that captures that moment:

I am healthy and vital.
My body is strong and graceful.
I have the confidence to achieve my goals.

These simple affirmations hold tremendous power to motivate change. Focus on that internal picture of yourself whenever you feel stressed or disheartened. Remind yourself of that image by writing down your affirmation, placing it where you are bound to see it often. It will act on your unconscious daily.

ART AS AFFIRMATION

An affirmation can be visual—artworks and images that surround you can inspire your thoughts and nourish your spirit. Use art as affirmation in your home, your office, even your car—anywhere you spend significant amounts of time.

In this society, we are surrounded by images that tell us how to look, think, behave, and how we should feel about ourselves. I suggest you create your own world, a world that affirms you and the majority of American women, by consciously choosing to incorporate other images and ideas enabling you to counterbalance what so many popular fashion magazines tell us is the ideal woman. Remember—there are millions of plus-size women who share your outlook and whose collective efforts are changing what it means to be a large woman today. Envision yourself as part of a larger movement of size acceptance with powerful affirmations!

I decorate my studio with Matisse reproductions, chosen because they convey the innate beauty of the human form and spirit. You might choose to decorate your living space with reproductions by artists such as Rubens, Frans Hals, Titian, Raphael, Goya, Botero, François Boucher, or sculptures by Henry Moore—even the voluptuous fertility goddess Venus of Willendorf. These images will serve as a reminder that throughout history our ample curves have been much admired and revered. You might wish to spend an afternoon wandering through an art museum and admiring voluptuous women in painting. In addition, many museums are online, including the famed Metropolitan Museum of Art and the Louvre. These Web sites afford you a chance to view their precious collections at leisure. Afterward, make a quick trip to their online gift shop and purchase the posters, greeting cards, and other items that validate you as a full-figured woman.

Because we are bombarded with images of what we are supposed to look like, it is especially important to create an environment with images of our choosing, images that validate us as real women and human beings. The images you choose need not be images of plus-size women. Rather, they may simply be images like those of Matisse, which convey the beauty and grace of the human spirit and show how the body is life itself. You may feel more comfortable with images of voluptuous women, or you may prefer images which are less body-specific, and more representational. It's up to you to decide which images validate you.

MUSICAL AFFIRMATIONS

They say that music is the language of the soul. Surely, more than almost any other medium, it has the power to transform your mood. Music is an important way of affecting your physical, emotional, and spiritual self, and it can work on the subconscious level as an affirmation. It's fascinating for me to watch women come alive in the studio with different styles of music. The secret is variety. It's as if the notes strike a chord deep within their souls. The music seems to beg the women to move, uniting rhythms with spirits. Whether it's classical, Motown, country, or swing, the uninhibited connection of music and movement is breathtaking to observe.

If you don't already incorporate music into your life, this may be the time to consider it—both as a tool for working out and as a means of uplifting your spirit. Treat yourself to the music of women such as Odetta, Laura Nyro, Celia Cruz, Martha Washington, Rosemary Clooney, Aretha Franklin, Patti LaBelle, Queen Latifah, Sarah Vaughan, or opera singers such as Jessye Norman and Sharon Sweet. Hearing these women's powerful and expressive voices as you move through your day, you access the power and wisdom of their words and song. They will help you to envision a self that is creative, expressive, active, and free.

Affirmations, in all their forms, are your most effective tool for living. They offer a wonderful mode of self-expression, can be inexpensive, and, best of all—they're incredibly effective. More than any book, health club membership, or expensive new gym outfit, affirmations of all dimensions will motivate you to movement as you embark on this program.

CHAPTER FOUR

CREATING SUPPORT

To receive everything, one must open one's hands and give.
—Taisen Deshimaru

When people put their minds to something the possibilities for transformation are endless. I have seen it time after time. So many of the women who walk through my doors undergo a marvelous transformation from despair to health and confidence. Of course, taking those first steps to living a life of movement and fitness can be daunting. Perhaps activity is so difficult that you shy away from attempting physical tasks, such as joining friends at a bowling alley or dancing at a wedding. The idea of working out, of course, seems overwhelming. You've purchased expensive workout equipment, but your treadmill acts as a clothes hanger, and your Thigh Master collects dust in the corner.

Perhaps the most dangerous by-product of the sedentary lifestyle is that inactivity becomes a sort of comfort zone; as long as you are physically inactive you don't have to be aware of your body, or consider the ways in which you may be disappointed with yourself. But it's a vicious cycle: You may have difficulty performing daily activities and suffer from aches and pains, so you limit your activities. By limiting your activities, they become even more difficult.

And so the downward cycle deepens. You are numbed, but the numbness is less threatening than the possibility of being more fully alive.

My client Jenny is a perfect example. A healthy woman for most of her life, she became less active when her husband left her after eight years of marriage. Jenny stopped going out socially, turned to food for solace, and added weight to a large frame. Occasionally, feeling guilty about having allowed herself to become so inactive, Jenny would sign up for a fitness class or attempt to work out on her own. But as Jenny discovered, the physical and the emotional realms are inextricably linked; just the act of moving her body made Jenny more aware of her feelings of sadness and loss and her anger toward her husband. Jenny was disappointed with herself for not taking better care of her body and spirit, but deep down she was afraid to do anything about it—she feared facing the feelings that movement would stir up. Eventually she stopped even trying to work out, since it seemed to make her more unhappy than before. She had become accustomed to numbing the pain.

Change is difficult, especially in the area of fitness. For women of size it is even more difficult, since one has to struggle with the dual challenges of self-motivation—an enormous struggle for anybody—and the poisonous messages from society about large bodies being unworthy of care. These messages, delivered in advertising, television, and the casual cruelty of everyday bigotry, act as a tremendous block on our motivation.

Jenny knew that to make the change from a sedentary lifestyle to an active one meant taking a psychological risk. She would have to be willing to face newly awakened feelings of discomfort and unhappiness. But she had finally reached a point where she was willing to try, and she did so by beginning the program in *Real Fitness for Real Women*.

Jenny was reluctant to tell too many people about the program because she didn't want to contend with other people's unrealistic expectations about weight loss. She enlisted her best friend Charlotte's support. Jenny felt she needed affirmation from at least one outside source—one person to offer support and encouragement. As it turns out, Charlotte, who hadn't attempted a fitness program in several years, agreed to join her for the six-week program. The women became excited about the prospect of getting fit. They ordered several workout outfits from a catalogue, and agreed to motivate each other on days when one or the other was thinking of quitting. By taking a risk, Jenny and Charlotte sowed the seeds of their success.

Of course, the first place to look for support is within. Since our society equates fitness with thinness, you may have a hard time validating your own desire to be fit. But once you abandon the preoccupation with body size and start to focus on how you feel on the inside, it is a lot easier to make that connection.

During your workouts, allow yourself to enjoy the way your body feels as you move through space. Savor the pleasure of being able to stretch further than you were able to last week, or do repetitions more easily. Even if it's only for 30 minutes each week, it's a time when you can abandon all stressful thoughts and know that you're doing something good for yourself. Move your body in ways you may not have allowed yourself since you were a child. Synchronize your movements to your favorite music, and allow the rhythms to swirl around you and move through you, quickening your step.

After our workouts we thank different parts of our bodies. Pour your love of your self and your appreciation of your body into those areas about which you feel positive. Focus on the parts that you like—soft, pretty hair, beautifully formed lips, artfully painted fingernails and toes. Perhaps you are proud of your cleavage, your strong calves, aspects of your curviness that feel comfortable and feminine. When you get dressed in the morning, highlight the areas you like best by wearing open-toed sandals, a flowing dress, or jewelry that draws attention to the hands. Revel in yourself!

The second place to look for support is through other people you already know, such as friends and family. Since plus-size women don't get that support from society at large—in fact, when we enter gyms we are often made to feel that we don't belong—our friends and family may be able to step in.

Families and loved ones can be a marvelous source of support. Anita, an educator raising two children, says her kids started working out with her so that exercise could become a family activity. And Chava gets support from her husband, who drives her to class and respects her need to feel better about herself.

Perhaps you have friends who struggle with some of the same issues and you could persuade them to join your fitness journey. Or you might register your name on our Web site at www.infitnessinhealth.com and discover whether there are other women with similar goals in your area. Whether you decide to meet with them or simply communicate by telephone or e-mail, it makes sense to share your struggle and hope. You are not alone!

Sisters Kathy and Peg joined the program together in order to support each other. In the beginning they always came together, calling each other at work and scheduling their classes at the same time. Whenever one of them felt her commitment lagging, the other would remind her how great she'd feel after working out. Finally, after many months, fitness became more of a habit, and each of the women began to feel secure enough about her commitment to her own health to come on her own.

The success of In Fitness & In Health is due to the safe and nurturing environment, where women can exercise physically and feel secure emotionally. To know that you are part of a community of women working toward the same goals is comforting, rewarding, and fulfilling. A facility like In Fitness & In Health may not be available in your area, which is why I've written *Real Fitness for Real Women*. Now you have the program so many women have successfully used to get fit. In order to motivate yourself more, you may want to replicate the class experience by sharing your progress and the program with other like-minded women. Working out together can be a lot of fun, provided the atmosphere remains supportive and free of judgment.

However, sometimes resistance comes from the unlikeliest places. If you choose to tell friends and family about your new plan of action, there may be those who seem less than supportive.

Ann reports that since she reestablished her commitment to fitness, relatives at family dinners scrutinize what she eats, almost as though they are expecting her to fail. When she reaches for another helping of food just like everybody else, they shake their heads or suck in their breath, as if to say, "Oh, she's back to her old ways!" Part of the reason for this kind of resistance is that people are often most comfortable with what they know. If your family knows you to be inactive, they balk at the idea that you might change. If they count on you to take care of their needs first and put your own needs last on the list, they may have trouble when you begin to make your own needs more of a priority.

What is the best way to deal with unsupportive friends and family? Sometimes ignoring their criticisms is the best course. If, however, you feel compelled to say something, try repeating this affirmative phrase: "I accept my size and I am getting fit." Faced with such a positive and self-confident statement, critics no longer have a toehold and are forced to evaluate why they are so quick to judge you. These people may unconsciously wish to sabotage your progress so that they won't have to examine their own demands and expectations.

A third place to look for support is through the size acceptance community. By bonding together, we create a positive movement toward self-satisfaction and self-acceptance, changing both ourselves and society. This is no longer a fat or thin issue—body acceptance is a *women's* issue.

The size acceptance movement works for a more embracing attitude toward people of size and fights for our rights. Many events, such as the yearly National Association to Advance Fat Acceptance convention, are a lot of fun, with speakers, parties, and workshops all tailored to people with your concerns.

If politicking isn't your style, you might want to get acquainted with some of the publications and Web sites that can help you connect with like-minded people all over the world. *MODE* magazine, which launched in 1997 and has a circulation of nearly one million, is a terrific fashion magazine serving "real-sized" women. I also highly recommend the magazines *Radiance* and *BBW: Big Beautiful Women*, which offer just the right balance of politics, entertainment news, opinions, and fashion. Another great magazine, *Belle*, focuses on the plus-size woman of color; and *Extra-Hip* and *Girl* are geared toward young women and teens. The Internet is a wonderful tool for connecting with other plus-size people. Web sites such as *Fat!So?* provide a great forum for large people, where you'll find everything from discussions of the health care system to critiques of the media. Another Web site called *Health At Any Size* offers a size-friendly network of health and fitness professionals. All of these resources are listed in the back of the book.

However you create support—be it internally, through the help of family and friends, or by making connections with other women of size—you will discover that every little bit of effort you make toward your physical well-being has a positive and immediate impact, not only for yourself but for all women. You join the community of those who prove to the world that fitness knows no size. Embodying fitness and health, you become a beacon of pride.

CHAPTER FIVE

EVALUATING YOUR CURRENT ABILITIES

Perfectionism is self-abuse of the highest order.
—Anne Wilson Schaef

Every woman comes to my studio with a unique set of physical and emotional needs. Not a single client who walks through my door can be labeled or classified; she is her own woman, with her own history and set of life circumstances. But in the course of participating in the program many women discover they share some common ground.

Many of you struggled with weight as children and adolescents. Perhaps you were shamed by your families or schoolmates, made to feel as though your body was unacceptable. Some of you suffered from illness or trauma, either physical or emotional, which had major repercussions in your lives. Or you may have spent your entire lives dieting to no avail, and despaired of ever finding a program that could help.

Most of the women I see have common physical ailments, which have been factored into the program. Some cannot sit down on or get up from a bench without assistance. Many suffer from lower back pain, joint discomfort, and improper posture. There may be fear and emotional insecurity surrounding their ability to begin the program. But while you may share some of the same challenges, there is no template. Your body, and your spirit, are uniquely yours.

You may, at some point in your life, have asked yourself, "How did I get here?" It's a complicated question, and one not easily answered. People come in all sizes. We don't have to explain why some people are taller than others, and we shouldn't have to explain why some people are heavier than others. Variety is a law of nature. Through my studies and my work, I have identified five theories that may contribute to being a woman of size. Understand that there is still little we know about all of this, and the following are some theories with varying degrees of data support.

GENETICS

Many of you are predisposed to having a larger frame and carrying more weight. If your ancestors were large, chances are you will be too. In fact, if both your parents are big, you have an eighty percent chance of being large yourself. People from certain countries or regions are genetically predisposed to being bigger. Scandinavians are generally taller and larger-boned than the French, for example.

It is important to recognize and accept your body type. Those of you who are naturally large know that even when you eat moderately your body instinctively maintains itself at a certain size or set point. To try to whittle yourself down to a size 8 or 10 would be to fight a difficult and losing battle. However, some naturally large people do manage to lose a lot of weight through crash diets or time-consuming athletic routines. Oprah Winfrey's highly publicized weight loss program was a regimen of early morning lengthy runs and weight training, plus a strict low-fat diet—all supervised by an on-call trainer. But many of us would like to be fit without undertaking Olympic training regimens, and prefer not to deprive ourselves of many of the foods we enjoy. You can get results without pushing yourself too far and without depriving yourself. Through my program, you'll learn how.

FAMILY ENVIRONMENT

Charmaine was a fairly picky eater as a child—there were certain foods, such as tomatoes, bananas, and fish, which she simply did not like. But her mother disregarded her preferences and required her to eat everything on her plate, saying she could not leave the dinner table otherwise. If, like Charmaine, you grew up in a family where you had to clean your plate, were forced to eat adult-sized portions, and had to finish everything you were served for dinner before you were allowed dessert, you are more likely to have developed a problem with weight.

Many cultures and communities, especially those once plagued by poverty, famine, or political instability, view the "robust child" as the ideal. In such families, it is often very important to have a complete meal on the table and for everyone to eat until all the food is gone. If you were encouraged to eat past the point of fullness, you didn't learn how to tune into your own body signals. If you were from one of these cultures or communities, you are likelier to have developed a problem with being overweight.

As a child, you may have been denied certain foods because your parents tried to control your weight. You developed cravings for those foods, and overate them to compensate for having been denied. The absence or denial of particular foods may interrupt the natural rhythm of the body. Food may then be used as a mood-altering substance or a self-soothing technique, a pattern that has stayed with you into adulthood.

HEALTH CONDITIONS

Many health factors and conditions contribute to the accumulation of weight. Sometimes the medications designed to treat certain conditions slow down the metabolism or throw off hormonal balance, which can result in weight gain. One of the common side effects of a medication for lupus causes people to put on weight. Certain antidepressants, hormone replacement therapy, and steroids prescribed for infections and other conditions tend to cause weight gain. If you have been in this situation you know how frustrating and pointless all the talk of losing weight can be.

Jamie was an average-sized woman who worked as a nurse in an intensive care unit and ran a farm with her husband. But when she discovered she had contracted lupus, she was forced to take drugs that slowed down her metabolism to a near standstill. In short order she gained 80 pounds. Jamie still lives with lupus. She has adjusted to her new body size and gives thanks for each day she is able to survive her disease.

Similarly, Ellen had gained some weight with each of her two children but maintained an active lifestyle and felt satisfied with her level of fitness. But a difficult twin pregnancy changed all that. After Ellen experienced contractions in her fifth month, her doctor put her on medication and ordered her to stay in bed for the remainder of her pregnancy. She developed diabetes and her weight snowballed. After the twins were born, Ellen had so many responsibilities at home there was little time to work out. Today Ellen wishes she were as fit and strong as she used to be.

There are many health reasons that could have caused you to put on weight. From a difficult pregnancy to surgery or injury, bodies react to a variety of situations by increasing stores of energy in the form of fat once physical activity is reduced. With illness, however, you could lose a significant amount of weight while the body tries to recover from the blow to the immune system. Whatever the health condition, speak with your doctor in depth to fully understand any significant weight loss or weight gain.

EMOTIONAL TRAUMA

Often an event with emotional impact has physical repercussions. Many of you can trace your weight gain to some traumatic event: divorce, violation, death of a loved one, loss of a job. You may have reacted to the trauma by becoming sedentary, putting up armor to protect you from further trauma, or by using food to manage your feelings of loss or anxiety. Sometimes women even react to the good things in life by gaining weight, almost as if to undercut their achievements or prevent themselves from realizing their good fortune.

A hard-hitting life event can be a turning point. Phyllis cared for her mother, who was sick with Alzheimer's, for many years. As her mother became more and more dependent on her, Phyllis no longer made her own health a priority. She stopped exercising, and instead of preparing herself healthy meals she grabbed fast food when she could or skipped meals, then binged at night to compensate for feelings of sadness and exhaustion.

Judy had reached the pinnacle of her television producing career at the young age of forty. Interviewing famous people while earning a six-digit income and displaying an Emmy award on her shelf were not in alignment with her loss of personal joy and freedom. Long work hours and a highly successful, image-demanding career had robbed Judy of her sense of self. Weight gain became the unwelcome measure of her success. The greatness and financial abundance of her career could not replace the dramatic self-care needed to balance her life.

Whether it is a positive or negative event in your life, if it affects you emotionally, you could experience weight gain while working through the issues. Acknowledge what is happening and seek appropriate care through health professionals and supportive family and friends.

INACTIVE LIFESTYLE

An inactive lifestyle is not healthful for anyone, regardless of size. Thin people often assume they don't have to work out, and larger people feel as if they can't. Both are mistaken. Exercise has been shown to prevent a myriad of debilitating conditions, from heart disease to high blood pressure to osteoporosis, and is even a factor in the prevention of cancer. An inactive lifestyle is more cause for alarm than being "overweight."

Studies by Dr. Steven N. Blair, director of research at the Cooper Institute for

Aerobics Research, prove that "the greatest reductions in premature death rates are achieved by getting totally unfit people to become just moderately fit. The men and women who stand to benefit the most are those going from nothing to something."

Paul Ernsberger and Paul Haskew note, in the *New England Journal of Medicine* (1986), that inadequate exercise and a lack of dietary fiber, along with excessive consumption of alcohol, fat, and sugar, will contribute to disease while promoting weight gain. And as Glenn A. Gaesser, Ph.D., writes in his book *Big Fat Lies*, "overcoming inertia must come from within." The focus, he suggests, should be placed on "physical activity" rather than exercise, with more emphasis placed on trying to get moving at any intensity.

All three experts agree that an inactive lifestyle may precipitate weight gain; however, a level of fitness at any weight is far more beneficial than a sedentary lifestyle.

DIETING

Unfortunately, as most of you have discovered, dieting doesn't lead to permanent weight loss, and usually doesn't make you healthy. In fact, it often has the reverse effect. Yo-yo dieting is one theory about why people gain weight over time and experience higher rates of heart disease. (Figures for higher heart disease rates among yo-yo dieters have been published in the Framingham Heart Study and the Multiple Risk Factor Intervention Trial. As Glenn Gaesser writes: "After more than three decades of follow-up evaluations that included biannual body weight measurements, those Framingham subjects whose body weights yo-yoed the most had up to a 100 percent greater risk of death from heart disease than those whose weights fluctuated the least!")

Many women who come to my program are products of two decades of the diet industry. From appetite suppressants to stomach stapling, they've been through it all. Whether it's a liquid diet, single food diet, or the Champagne and Lollipop diet, all are guaranteed to disrupt the natural state of the body in all its glory. The temporary joy of weight loss may give way to disastrous heartache once the weight returns. Diets that prescribe under 1200 calories a day use up not only fat but muscle tissue for fuel. However, weight is put back on in the form of fat and water. Fat acceptance activist Lynn McAfee is a prime example. At age ten, when her family expressed concern about her large frame, her family doctor prescribed diet drugs. Today, weighing in at 500 pounds, she says she has dieted her way up the scale. You may feel that you too have been a slave to the bathroom scale, only to realize that dieting doesn't lead to permanent weight loss.

Whatever your history, however you have arrived at where you are today, it is important to understand that weight gain does not make you any less acceptable of being fit or any less worthy as a human being. You may or may not be happy with your size, but at no size are you incapable of becoming physically fit and improving your health. If you have felt as though you were too out of shape to qualify for any of the fitness programs out there, the program in *Real Fitness for Real Women* is for you. Similarly, if you are a large woman who is active and fit, this program will help you take your degree of physical awareness and fitness to a new level by offering techniques designed specifically for you.

While I do not subscribe to weighing, measuring, or other sorts of standardized testing, I encourage women to evaluate themselves and rate their own fitness level in order to set goals. The following questionnaire will help you assess your current level of fitness. There are no right or wrong answers; this is merely a tool to help you determine where you are today.

ASSESSMENT QUESTIONNAIRE FOR FUNCTIONAL FITNESS

Answer these 12 questions before you begin your program and then again at the end of the six weeks. This questionnaire is based on the introductory program I designed and incorporate in my studio. I am certain you will notice an increase in your Activities of Daily Living (ADLs) and quality of life at the end of the program!

1. When you climb a flight of stairs, do you hold on to the railing?
   a. Never (3)
   b. Sometimes (2)
   c. Always (1)

2. Do you have to stop and rest when climbing a flight of stairs (approximately 15 steps)?
   a. Never (3)
   b. Sometimes (2)
   c. Always (1)

3. When you walk a block or two are you able to carry on a conversation?
   a. Never (1)
   b. Sometimes (2)
   c. Always (3)

4. Do you become easily fatigued when you exercise or move your body?
   a. Never (3)
   b. Sometimes (2)
   c. Always (1)

5. Do you sleep through the night without interruption?
   a. Never (1)
   b. Sometimes (2)
   c. Always (3)

6. In a seated position, are you able to bend over and tie your shoes?
   a. Never (1)
   b. Sometimes (2)
   c. Always (3)

7. Are you able to get in and out of the bathtub to take a bath without assistance?
    a. Never (1)
    b. Sometimes (2)
    c. Always (3)

8. Are you able to get up from the floor without assistance?
    a. Never (1)
    b. Sometimes (2)
    c. Always (3)

9. Are you able to climb on a chair or stepladder?
    a. Never (1)
    b. Sometimes (2)
    c. Always (3)

10. Do you have persistent lower back pain and/or joint stiffness?
    a. Never (3)
    b. Sometimes (2)
    c. Always (1)

11. How would you rate your energy level?
    a. Low (1)
    b. Moderate (2)
    c. High (3)

12. Are you able to complete 20 minutes of continuous movement?
    a. Never (1)
    b. Sometimes (2)
    c. Always (3)

Add up your scores.

36 points: Congratulations! You are leading a Full and Active Lifestyle. Master the techniques in this book and consider passing this book on to a friend who may also benefit.

24–35 points: Maintaining an Active Lifestyle. You are moving in your life and seem to incorporate well many of the ADLs in question. Have you overcome social barriers with regards to exercise—the program's highest achievement? Try a company bowling party or a fund-raising walk for breast cancer or diabetes. If you haven't already done so, move your movement to the outside world!

13–23 points: Developing an Active Lifestyle. You are still working on understanding your body and its function with regard to daily activities. Master the connection from the muscles to the brain so a clear signal can be repeated until the correct response is learned.

0–12 points: Introduction to an Active lifestyle. This book is the best place for you to start. While it may seem difficult and overwhelming at times, remember to build your program slowly based on function as opposed to weight loss.

CHAPTER SIX

GETTING STARTED

Discipline doesn't have to be about restrictions, it can be about freedom. . . it can be about more rather than less.

—Bhatya Zumir

As with any new journey or endeavor, embarking on a fitness program requires a bit of advance planning. While you may be so flush with motivation that you want to jump up and start moving immediately, there are a few things to keep in mind. The exercise program in *Real Fitness for Real Women* requires some special equipment, as listed below:

◆ Water
◆ Bath towel
◆ Dynaband: a four-foot balloon-like latex band, available in varying degrees of resistance
◆ Free weights (optional): one- to three-pound dumbbells
◆ Armless chair
◆ STEP bench (optional): a bench approximately three and a half feet long and four inches high, which comes with four two-inch blocks

✦ Exercise mat (optional)
✦ 8 1/2-inch playground ball or bed pillow
✦ Music

Where to purchase this equipment is listed in the Resources section in the back of this book. Before beginning you should be mindful of proper skin care and foot care issues specific to women of size. You'll also need to secure a supply of workout clothing that will make your exercise sessions as pleasant and beneficial as possible.

I offer the professional expertise of three highly respected specialists who have worked with plus-size women and their unique concerns. Dr. Laurie Polis, one of the nation's leading dermatologists, offers comprehensive information about skin care. Dr. Sherri Greene, a holistic podiatrist with a thriving Manhattan business, gives pointers on how to avoid common foot ailments. And Anne Kelley, president of Junonia, a five-year-old activewear company that caters to large women, offers basic recommendations for choosing workout clothes.

SKIN CARE

When it comes to movement and fitness, plus-size women have unique skin care concerns. Chafing is probably the number one problem; repetitive movements, combined with working up a sweat, can cause skin to rub against skin, producing discomfort and pain.

Fortunately, one can guard against chafing with minimal effort. But contrary to popular belief, using baby power is not one of them. Many of you probably use baby powder to protect against chafing in your daily life. However, when you're working out, leave the talcum powder in the medicine cabinet. Sure, a liberal sprinkling may feel wonderful for the first ten minutes. But the last thing you need is lumps of wet powder collecting in your skin folds. Better to protect against skin rubbing skin with the proper clothing.

Chafing can occur with different degrees of severity; many cases result in no more than a minor irritation, but I have seen skin that has been rubbed raw and is exquisitely tender. When chafing does occur, it should be treated immediately to avoid worsening the problem. You can treat a case of chafed skin with ice packs and the same ointments you use for diaper rash. If severe chafing occurs, it is best to stop exercising for a few days and rethink what you are wearing. Women who do a lot of stationary cycling are prone to chafing on the inner thighs. If this occurs, switch to upper body or floor work for a change.

Your face and body may become flushed and reddish in your skin's attempt to regulate your temperature. For this reason, it is best to avoid cover-up make-up—your skin needs to breathe freely. Lip gloss or balm, however, is a good idea, because it helps prevent drying out the skin on your lips. Moisturizer is absolutely unnecessary. Pores should remain open and expressive.

One way to keep your body comfortable as you work out is to exercise in a ventilated area. If you are in a room where the air is stagnant, or if it is a hot and muggy day, I suggest using a fan to circulate the air.

Hormones and metabolism are affected by activity level. As you begin to work out your body may go through hormonal changes, causing acne break-outs. Eruptions often occur on the hairline, the buttocks, the thighs, or the back. If your acne becomes severe you may wish to consult a dermatologist. But over-the-counter medications can also treat the problem.

To prevent acne of the face, stock up on clean broad white cotton bands to absorb the sweat that appears at your hairline. The choice of white is not just a fashion statement—white is good because colored dyes can bleed out as you sweat. Also, darker colors are generally more allergenic, and lighter colors retain less heat. You might also wish to invest in several pairs of cotton wrist-bands. When you perspire heavily and sweat starts to get in your eyes, try not to wipe it away with your hands, which may carry dirt or oils. Instead, you can keep your eyes clear and your skin clean by dabbing the sweat away with your sweatbands.

If you use an anti-acne medication on your face, don't put it above your eyes before a workout because as you perspire it may drip into your eyes.

After your workout, remove your workout clothes. If you allow your sweat to stay next to your skin too long, you can develop acne, latex/rubber allergies, or dermatitis.

Showering helps prevent superficial yeast infections. Yeast loves to grow in warm, moist, skin-touching-skin places, and especially thrives when the body temperature is high. It's also best to purchase enough workout outfits to enable you to wear clean clothes each time. Yeast loves body folds—the belly, under the breasts, and the area where the thighs meet the torso. In the shower, you might want to use an antibacterial soap on body folds.

Dry off carefully after you shower, and pay attention to the body folds. It may take more time and energy to see that you are really dry, but it is worth it, as allowing moisture to linger is asking for trouble.

While you are working out, avoid costume jewelry because it can be irritating to the skin. Perspiration can cause the nickel in costume jewelry to leech out, causing dermatitis.

Lastly, working out outside can be a lot of fun—but don't forget the sunscreen!

FOOT CARE

Dr. Greene recommends shopping for a good running shoe regardless of the type of exercise you prefer. Running shoes, as opposed to cross-trainers or walking shoes, offer the most support. Spend some time trying on different styles; you might want to look for one with extra width. Make sure there is adequate room in the toe box, so your foot isn't crowded and compressed.

It's important to keep toenails on the shorter side. When you begin to work out, increased pressure on the foot can result in toe box problems if nails curl down and irritate the toe.

Women of size are prone to a number of foot conditions, including heel spur syndrome. This is a painful condition that occurs in the heel due to excess pulling of the plantar fascia—a fibrous tissue network that extends from the base of the toes to the heel bone. The added pulling creates an inflammation process, which forms the spur. You can prevent heel spur syndrome by stretching and strengthening the muscles for the lower leg, as demonstrated in Chapter 7 (see Week 4).

If you do develop heel spur syndrome, ice your feet every day for a few days (twenty minutes of icing every hour). Continue to stretch the feet slowly. Restrict your activity. If the pain continues, seek podiatric care. The podiatrist may prescribe an anti-inflammatory for the heel spur. (Note: Two all-natural anti-inflammatories are Bromelian and Boswellia.)

Corns seem to afflict almost every woman, but they are especially common among plus-size women, who may have trouble finding shoes that fit correctly. A corn is caused by a deformity of the bone. It can also be hereditary or exacerbated by tight shoes. The body responds to pressure by forming a layer of protective skin over the joint. Corns can either be treated conservatively, by removing the layer of dead skin and putting a protective shield on the toe, or aggressively, by surgically treating the underlying bone.

Women of size may have flat feet due to overpronation (rolling in). This stresses the Achilles tendon and can cause conditions such as Achilles tendinitis, an inflammation of the long cord at the back of the heel. Achilles tendinitis is not only caused by poor biomechanics such as pronating, but also by overuse or trauma. Dr. Greene treats this condition by prescribing an anti-inflammatory and a program of stretching, physical therapy, and food adjustments to assist in healing. Most important is prevention: making sure the foot is functioning as it should, avoiding overpronating, and ensuring that shoes have adequate arch support or orthotics specific to you. The program in *Real Fitness for Real Women* will train you in proper body mechanics, going a long way to avoiding the development of such disorders.

CLOTHING

Only five years ago, there wasn't much in the way of activewear for women of size. Today, companies such as Junonia and Plus Woman offer attractive, stylish workout wear. Junonia carries styles in sizes up to 6X, and Plus Woman makes clothing to order.

Your exercise clothing should be something you enjoy putting on. It will cheer you up, give you positive affirmation to take better care of yourself, and put you in the right frame of mind for your workouts. Regard your workout clothing as a uniform and treat it with care and respect. If you don't feel comfortable in your workout clothes, it may be very emotionally difficult to exercise around others or even go for a walk around the block. Wearing clothing you like will make you feel better about overcoming social barriers with regards to exercise.

The importance of a woman's fitness apparel should not be minimized. It is better to start off with clothing you love, which maximizes your comfort, so you can get the most out of your workouts—physically and psychologically—right now. Many women of size make uninformed choices about activewear due to lack of knowledge.

You may be self-conscious at first about revealing your body and choose big T-shirts and other cover-ups. But if you're heavy, it's important to have the kind of clothing that protects skin from rubbing against skin. It may be better to wear clothing that is somewhat form-fitting so that the body folds are covered and protected.

Another poor choice is loose, baggy sweatpants. Sweatpants can be very comfortable in the winter, but in warmer months they keep you overheated, and they do little to protect the skin from chafing. It's better to wear leggings or shorts (or anything in between) that you feel comfortable in.

Sports bras are important for support and motion control. Cotton sports bras may feel good and offer sufficient support for low-impact activities such as gardening, walking, or biking, but for the next level of activity, such as aerobics or court sports, you should choose a more structured athletic bra. The sports bra will make the breasts feel like they are pressed into your chest.

It's particularly important to wear clothing that wicks away sweat so that you can cool down as fast as your body is able. Fat cells have a lot of water in them, and plus-size women can sweat copiously. These days there are a myriad of highly specialized sports fabrics, which can really make a difference in how you feel in your clothing. Cotton absorbs and holds sweat, but does not wick it away from your skin. Cotton may be a good fabric if you are able to change right after a workout, but it's not optimal if you plan to exercise over a longer period of time. Junonia makes clothing out of a trademarked fabric called Quikwik, a fiber that dries while you wear it. Other synthetics such as Coolmax keep you cooler by wicking your sweat away from your skin. It makes sense to give a few things a try and discover what works best for you.

OTHER WORKOUT TIPS

There's nothing like your favorite CD or cassette to motivate you to swing your arms and move your hips. If you have not incorporated music into your life until now, here's your chance to explore what you like. Purchase several cassettes of music you enjoy, and play them during your workouts. For the breathing sections you may prefer music that's calm or hypnotic; for stretching and aerobics, faster, up-tempo music does the trick. Don't feel as though you have to listen to the kind of music you usually hear in aerobics studios, however—it's important to choose music you truly enjoy. (There are aerobic music company recommendations in the Resources section.) Whether you prefer dance music, country and western, or jazz standards, your selection will help you form positive associations with exercise and keep your workout fun and exciting.

It's a good idea to work out in the same place, so you develop a sense of routine. In this way, fitness becomes second nature, a positive habit.

Finally, keep in mind that fitness is not an "all or nothing" venture. You don't have to work out every single day to be fit—once a week is a successful beginning to maintain an active lifestyle. (Dr. Steven N. Blair recommends walking two minutes a day to begin!) If you miss one week or get out of the habit, don't beat yourself up. You haven't failed—just fallen out of practice. It's important to maintain a gentle attitude of self-support and self-love.

CHAPTER SEVEN

THE PROGRAM

Bit by bit . . . she had claimed herself. Freeing herself was one thing;
claiming ownership of that freed self was another.
—Toni Morrison

At the core of *Real Fitness for Real Women* is the six-week introductory program, which has been used successfully in my studio. The six-week program helps women to reconnect with their bodies and understand that movement can be safe, fun, and healthy, rather than a punishing, "no pain no gain"experience. Many of the women who come to my studio for the first time are struggling with the fact that their minds have become profoundly disconnected from their bodies. My goal is to unite them.

The format of each week includes a warm-up, aerobics, strength training and stretching techniques, and meditation. Each week progresses incrementally, until you are able to sustain an aerobics session of 20 minutes. The reason we begin slowly is this: Many women have experienced unrealistic goals in traditional gyms, only to have failed again. We begin once a week to set accessible and achievable goals. If you feel motivated to work out more than once a week, feel free to do so, but keep in mind that this is a lifestyle change, not an overnight quick fix. Small gains build a foundation for long-term success.

Any aerobic movement (movement sustained for a minimum of twenty minutes) such as walking, dancing, and swimming can be performed on subsequent
days. The exercises in this book can be performed on a daily basis until the body
learns and understands the movement. I suggest you begin with the once-a-
week regimen for two reasons. The first is to keep your motivation up so you
don't get bored with your routine. The second reason is that you are building a
foundation for a lifetime. As with wealth accumulation for retirement, it's the
long-term investment that reaps the reward.

You will find some of the exercises, like the Lower Back Stretch or The Wave,
offer immediate relief to aches and pains. You can add these to a daily routine
if you would like. To increase the challenge of the program, you may incorporate resistance with free weights, or increase the intensity. There are notes on
each of the exercises to explain how this can be done.

Each week is divided into four sections. Section I is the Warm-up, followed
by Section II, Your Personal Aerobic Program. Section III is Strength Training
and Stretching Techniques. Each week is completed with a Meditation in
Section IV. Choose one day a week as your official exercise day to become part
of your weekly routine. Monday is a great day to formally begin your workout
because you are starting the week afresh, filled with hope and determination.
Exercising on Monday will put you in the right frame of mind for the rest of the
week. But if Monday isn't a good day for you, choose any day that works, being
sure to consistently work out on that day.

I ask you to keep the Warm-up the same each week so that your body will
start to incorporate biomechanical adaptation or muscle memory. With muscle
memory, more focus is on the movement instead of worrying about the choreography. The program consists of 25 exercises designed exclusively for your
body. While a fitness repertoire can be much more extensive, mastering these
25 specific exercises will prepare your body to experience all movement with
more joy and less pain—physically and emotionally. My experience has been
that after women complete Week 1 and master the Breathing for Me technique,
they say, "That's it?" Yes, that's it. Trust me, your breath is fuller, your cells are
ecstatic, your nervous system is well stimulated, and your mind is elated at the
idea of completing a successful session of fitness. You are well on your way to

reconnecting with your body in a way that serves you rather than destroys you. Enjoy the process. It is truly transforming.

WEEK ONE: BREATHING FOR ME
Theme for the Week: Mindful Movement

Goals:
1. Understand and master the Breathing for Me technique.
2. Connect your breath with your movement.

Exercises:
Section I ✦ Warm-up
Section II ✦ Your Personal Aerobic Program—First 5 Minutes
Section III ✦ Strength Training and Stretching Techniques
    1. Breathing for Me
    2. Knee to Chest Stretch
    3. Tilt and Bridge
    4. Pec Stretch
    5. Lower Back Stretch
Section IV ✦ Meditation

Equipment:
1. Mat for the floor (optional)
2. Towel and pillow
3. 8 1/2-inch playground ball
4. Music
5. Water

SECTION I: WARM-UP

(The Warm-up will be repeated each week)

✦ Inhale deeply, raising your arms up to the ceiling; then exhale, lowering your arms to your sides. Repeat 4 times.

✦ Roll your shoulders back 4 times.

✦ Roll your shoulders forward 4 times.

✦ Keeping the arms straight, lift the right arm up and back in a wide circle, as though doing the backstroke, then with the left. Complete 4 times.

✦ Circle the arms forward as if you were doing the crawl. Repeat 4 times.

✦ Push arms forward and then out to the sides as though doing the breast-stroke. Repeat 4 times.

✦ With the left hand on the hip and the right arm high, bend to the left side and stretch. Alternate right and left sides 4 times.

✦ Step forward on your right foot, bending the knee slightly. Stretch your left leg straight behind you, gently pressing the heel to the floor. You should feel a stretch in the left calf. Rest your hands on your right thigh or hold on to a chair or the wall for balance. Hold for 30 seconds, then change sides.

Throughout the arm sequence, the feet pattern remains the same by shifting the weight from side to side, maintaining a wide parallel position. While doing this:

✦ Reach the right arm up to the ceiling, then the left arm, then the right and left again. Reach the right arm across the chest, then the left, then right and left again. Repeat the sequence 4 times.

✦ Push both arms out to the left, then right, then left and right again. Reach both arms up to the ceiling on the left diagonal, then right, then left and right again. Repeat the sequence 4 times.

✦ Backstroke with the right arm, then left, then right and left again. Push the arms forward 4 times. Repeat the sequence 4 times.

✦ Bend the elbows up to the left, then right, then left and right again. Punch both arms out to the left, then right, then left and right again. Repeat the sequence 4 times.

SECTION II: YOUR PERSONAL AEROBIC PROGRAM—FIRST 5 MINUTES

First, put your music on and begin with a side-to-side step-touch. A step has weight and a touch has no weight. For example, step on the right foot (with weight) and touch the left foot (no weight). Your left foot should now be free to step left and touch right (no weight). Repeat continuously. You will begin to feel your circulation increase as you step-touch in time to the music. You can vary your aerobic routine by adding our walk-it-up combination. Starting on the right foot, take three steps forward, touch left, then take three steps back, touch right, all in time to the music. If you like you may also march in place, or add other dance moves you feel comfortable with. Pretend you are at a nightclub, boogying to the music. Continue for five minutes. Remember: It doesn't matter how fast you move—it's more important to keep moving.

SECTION III: STRENGTH TRAINING AND STRETCHING TECHNIQUES

The Breathing for Me technique is the base of this program. This breathing exercise is actually a form of strength training that will help firm up your abs. A strong abdominal wall decreases lower back discomfort, assists in climbing stairs, and decreases the risk of injury when lifting heavy objects. Strong abdominal muscles are the foundation for proper movement and correct body alignment.

Although we use our abdominal muscles all the time, many of us are not really sure where they are located, or how to strengthen them. There are four sets of abdominal muscles, and they span the area from the breastbone (sternum) to the pubic bone, attaching at different places on the ribs and pelvis. The following exercise will help you locate and tone the abdominal muscles. With all of the strength training exercises in *Real Fitness for Real Women*, success is achieved when the resting tone of your muscles increases. By that I mean you will actually begin to feel your muscles even while waiting in line at the bank or grocery store.

1. BREATHING FOR ME (ABDOMINALS)

Start Position

1. Sit forward on the edge of the chair with your feet resting comfortably flat on the floor. Lengthen your spine. Your back should be away from the back of the chair.

2. Your feet should be open at about the width of the chair legs.

3. Sit tall in the chair looking straight ahead ("eyes on the horizon").

The Exercise

1. While seated, begin to notice your breath. Keep this simple. Note that as you inhale, your abdominal wall expands, and when you exhale, the abdominal wall falls or softens.

2. Place both hands on your abdomen below your navel. Your fingertips should be pointing toward your pubic bone. Sitting in the start position, inhale, allowing your abdomen to expand forward into your hands.

3. As you exhale, gently use your hands to pull your abdominal (stomach) muscles UP and IN, as if you were zipping up a pair of pants.

4. Repeat 4 times, then rest by relaxing the abdominal muscles and maintaining the length of the spine.

5. Begin again, performing the exercise for another set of 4, and rest.

6. Repeat this exercise twice a day at your office desk, or any other time or place that is convenient. Repeat at least 2 times daily for the first week of the program.

Technique Moment

As you start to inhale, you may notice that you want to pull the abdominals in at the same time. We are erroneously taught to hold in our stomachs as we breathe in, which is incorrect. If you have trouble finding your natural breathing pattern, watch someone while they sleep. You will see that the natural pattern of breathing is to expand the abdomen as you inhale, and soften or pull in the abdomen as you exhale.

I cannot stress enough the importance of proper breathing techniques—breath is the key to life. We are increasing the awareness first, then working the muscles for support. But don't get discouraged if proper breathing techniques take a while to master. The natural rhythm is already within you. You may not have used it for some time, but this exercise will begin to get you back in touch with your breath and your body.

Once you have become more aware of your abdominals, you will no longer need to place your hands on your abdomen to perform this exercise, and you'll see that it can be performed anywhere! Ordinary moments such as driving or sitting at the desk or table are wonderful opportunities to work your abs.

Women who have had a cesarean section or other abdominal surgery may find it takes a little longer to master this exercise because scar tissue can inhibit some of the sensitivity in the abdominal region. Be patient and gentle with yourself—with practice and dedication you will soon feel the effects of stimulating your abdominal muscles.

The Breathing for Me technique can also be done on the floor. Simply follow the directions above while lying on the floor in the position shown on page 50.

Working with the same breathing techniques, the following exercises are designed to begin to connect your breath with your movement. Women of size often develop lower back pain because of the spill-out position—standing without utilizing abdominal support, and hence allowing the abdominals to "spill out." Muscles of the back hurt because they are not strong enough to do the work. Ideally, you want to be able to share the workload between the abdominal and back muscles.

The Knee to Chest Stretch and Tilt should begin to alleviate lower back discomfort. While performing these exercises, you may actually feel some discomfort in the lower back. A dull ache is fine—but any sharp, shooting pains mean you should discontinue the exercise immediately.

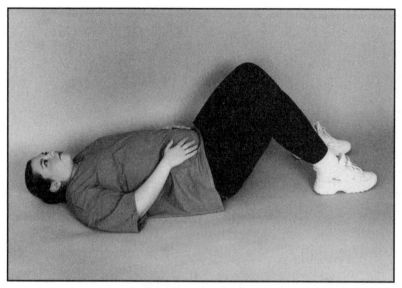

Breathing for Me (A)

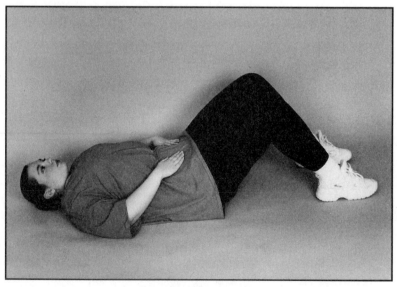

Breathing for Me (B)

2. KNEE TO CHEST STRETCH (QUADRATUS LUMBORUM)

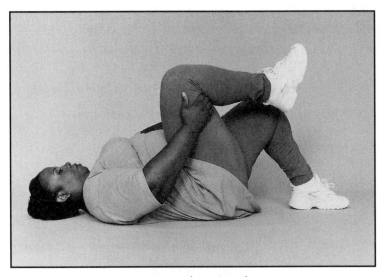

Knee to Chest Stretch

Start Position

On the floor or the bed, lie on your back and bend your knees. Feet should be flat on the floor or bed, hip width apart.

The Exercise

1. Bring the right knee to the chest, clasping your hands behind the thigh. If this is difficult, place a towel behind the thigh to assist you. If you feel your abdomen is in the way, turn the thigh out slightly.

2. Inhale and expand the abdominal wall like a balloon.

3. As you exhale, slowly draw the thigh to your chest. Repeat 4 times. Do the same with the left knee.

*Note that in most cases where multiple photographs are used to demonstrate an exercise, (A) illustrates the start position and (B) illustrates some midpoint movement, typically the position at which the muscles are flexed or under stress; one repetition is completed when the body returns to the start position.

3. TILT (ABS) AND BRIDGE (GLUTEALS AND HAMSTRINGS)

Start Position

Same as Knee to Chest Stretch.

The Exercise

1. Place ball between the thighs and rest your arms by your sides.
2. Inhale and expand the abdominal wall like a balloon.

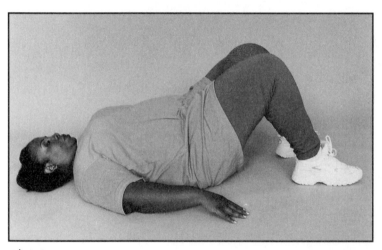

Tilt (A)

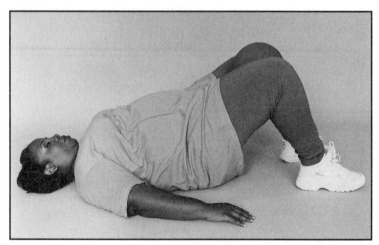

Tilt (B)

3. As you exhale, bring the navel to the spine, tighten the buttocks, and curl the tailbone off the floor, pressing the lower back into the floor or bed.

4. Use the abdominals to bring the pubic bone to the navel, instead of pressing the feet.

5. Inhale, and return to the start position.

6. Exhale and repeat 8 to 12 times.

Technique Moment

Women tend to lift their hips too high for this exercise. Be certain to breathe correctly and only lift the tailbone while rounding the lower back into the floor.

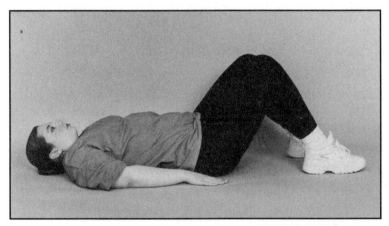

Bridge (A)

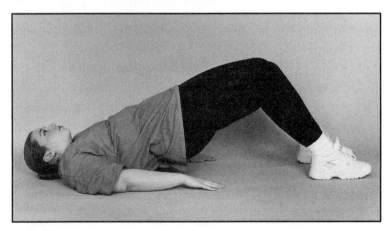

Bridge (B)

Proceed slowly. It takes time to build good technique. You may feel the back and the thighs (hamstrings) tighten. If you get a muscle cramp, stop for a moment. If you wish to increase the intensity and strengthen the back, try Bridges. The start position is the same as for Tilts but now lift the pelvis up to a 45-degree angle by pressing into the feet as shown in the photo. Hold for a count of ten, then lower slowly and repeat 4 times.

Finish today's workout with a Pec Stretch for the upper body and a Lower Back Stretch. Both are gentle stretches.

4. PEC STRETCH (PECTORALIS MAJOR)

Start Position
Same as Tilt, but with arms open in a V shape.

The Exercise
1. The pecs (pectoralis major) run from the breastbone (sternum) to the shoulders. Still on your back, open your arms to a V with palms facing the ceiling.
2. Inhale, expanding the abdominal wall.
3. As you exhale, bring the navel to the spine and allow your shoulders to relax into the floor. You may feel a slight stretch on the front of the shoulder. If it's too tight, put pillows under your arms.

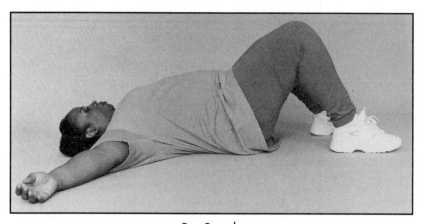

Pec Stretch

5. LOWER BACK STRETCH

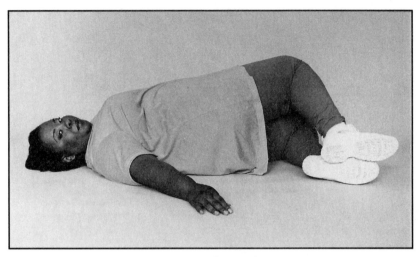

Lower Back Stretch

Start Position

Same as Pec Stretch, but with palms facing down, hands at waist level.

The Exercise

1. With thighs together, allow the knees to roll to the left, and roll your head to the right.
2. Inhale and exhale 4 times.
3. On the last exhale, bring your thighs back to the center.
4. Repeat on the right side.

Technique Moment

You are in control of the movement. Use the abdominals to control the rotation, and don't allow the legs to drop. If this is difficult, put a pillow under your thighs when your legs roll to the side. Continue with breathing technique.

SECTION IV: MEDITATION

Meditation is a tool for slowly reconnecting you with your body. After you have completed the exercises, sit quietly with your eyes closed. While you are in this relaxed state, focus on one part of your body that you like. It could be your eyes, your feet, or your fingernails. Stay focused on that part of your body for a few minutes. If negative thoughts come to mind, allow them to pass—picture yourself standing on a bridge and watching the negative thoughts float harmlessly downstream. After several minutes open your eyes and slowly stand up.

D A I L Y   F O C U S

Every week, for the days that you don't exercise, I offer an assignment for that day, represented by a key word or phrase. Each week the daily focus is the same, so that the daily reminders become a weekly habit. Amendments have been made for you if Monday is not your workout day.

Monday — MOVE!

On your workout days, enjoy the new sensations of moving your body. If this is not your workout day, consider adding some other form of movement, like climbing a flight of stairs or parking the car farther away from the store.

Tuesday — TRUE!

Be true and kind to yourself today. Ask yourself: How does my body feel after yesterday's movement? Forget the "no pain no gain" theory. The goal of yesterday's movement was not to make you sore. You may experience some slight muscle stiffness, but you should feel rejuvenated and energetic. Whether your workout day is Monday or not, pay attention to how you're breathing, and observe how you use specific muscle groups. If you feel stressed at any point during the day, remember to exhale. Conscious breathing will instantly decrease your stress level.

Wednesday — *WATER!*

Today we focus on water—the best health tonic in the world. Try to drink at least four eight-ounce glasses of water during the day. (Over the course of the program, work your way up to eight to ten.) Water washes away harmful internal toxins, keeps your skin looking young, and gives your body the energy it needs to function at peak level.

Thursday — *THINK!*

Think about how you can incorporate this program into your activities of daily living. Notice how you hold your body when you get up from chairs, desks, and even toilet seats. The modified squat exercise you learn in week 3 will provide you with good technique for performing these functional fitness activities.

Friday — *FRUITS and VEGETABLES!*

Today, incorporate more fresh fruits and vegetables into your meals. If it's time for a snack, reach for a pear or a bag of baby carrots. Enjoy the taste and texture of this marvelous "fast food."

Saturday — *SATISFIED!*

Today, satisfy the child within you by heading for the great outdoors. Ask a friend to join you for a walk, take your kids to the park, or go for a bike ride.

Sunday — *SPIRIT!*

Relax and reflect on your week. Give thanks for all the work you have done. Congratulations! You have laid the foundation for success.

WEEK TWO: ABSOLUTE ABS
Theme for the Week: Personal Power

Goals:
1. Move for 10 minutes.
2. Develop awareness of your muscles.
3. Understand correct abdominal work.

Exercises:
Section I ✦ Warm-up
Section II ✦ Your Personal Aerobic Program—Second 5 Minutes
Section III ✦ Strength Training and Stretching Techniques
     6. Superwoman
     7. The Wave
     8. Ball Squeeze
     9. Abs on the Incline
Section IV ✦ Meditation

Equipment:
1. Mat for the floor (optional)
2. Chair
3. 8 1/2-inch playground ball
4. STEP (optional) or pillow
5. Music
6. Water

SECTION I: WARM-UP

Today we begin the movement section with the same Warm-up as last week. I like to call it muscle memory—by repeating the same movements each week, the mind does not have to worry about learning complicated new choreography each time.

SECTION II: YOUR PERSONAL AEROBIC PROGRAM—SECOND 5 MINUTES

Once you've completed the Warm-up, put on the same piece of music you used last week and begin your Second 5 Minutes by repeating the routine from the First 5 Minutes in Week 1. Again, keep in mind that the goal is to keep moving—not to perform complex choreography. Add a second piece of music today, such as a pop or country and western tune. You are designing your own movement routine, so be sure to pick music that will continue to inspire you. If you wish, you may add the following choreography:

The Grapevine is a very common dance and aerobic step. Step to the side with the right foot, cross behind with the left, step to the side again with the right, and touch your left foot lightly next to the right. Keep in mind that a touch means you don't place your weight on that foot—you place it there only to pick it up again and continue with the sequence. Step to the left with the left foot, step behind with the right, step out on the left, and touch the right foot next to the left. If you wish, you may clap when you touch.

Leg Curls can also be added to your routine. Bring the right heel toward the right buttock (bending the leg back behind you) and then transfer the weight to the right foot. Alternate the legs and add arm movements by either pushing the arms forward, as if pushing someone away from you, to the side, or up, as if lifting luggage into an overhead bin. Let this movement be fun and playful.

Knee Lifts will begin to accelerate your heart rate, increasing the fresh supply of blood to all parts of the body. Imagine yourself as a marching soldier and lift the knees as high as you comfortably can. To improve your technique, master the Knee to Navel Connection. Each time you lift your knee, pull your navel in toward your spine. Alternate Grapevines, Leg Curls, and Knee Lifts until you complete your second five minutes.

SECTION III: STRENGTH TRAINING AND STRETCHING TECHNIQUES

6. SUPERWOMAN

Start Position
Place both hands on a sturdy chair seat with feet hip-width apart.

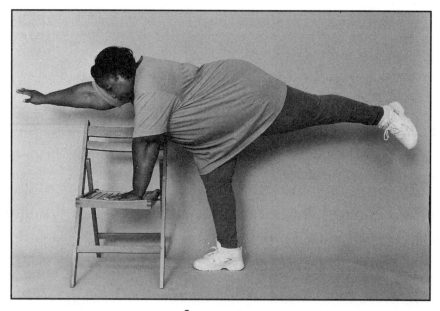

Superwoman

The Exercise

1. Keeping your abdominals strong, actively reach your right arm forward and your left leg back. Make yourself longer (pretend you are flying like Superwoman!). Right arm and left leg should be straight and elongated while parallel to the floor.

2. Reach for 4 counts and lower your limbs.

3. Reach left arm forward and right leg back. Hold for 4 counts and lower.

4. Repeat the entire sequence 4 to 8 times.

Technique Moment

The abdominals need to be held tight to keep the lower back from arching. If you experience any pain in the lower back, lower the leg and arm until you develop more strength. To increase the intensity, try adding a one-pound free weight (or a can of soup) in each hand.

7. THE WAVE

I developed this exercise for a client who regularly experienced lower back discomfort. She found that it helped her enormously.

Start Position

Sit in a sturdy chair with your feet turned out at a 45-degree angle, the knees pointing in the same direction as the feet. Your knees should be bent at a 90-degree angle.

The Exercise

1. Inhale, rocking forward on the pelvis, eyes to the ceiling.

2. As you exhale, round the chin into the neck and bring the navel to the spine.

3. Inhale and return to start position.

4. Repeat 4 times.

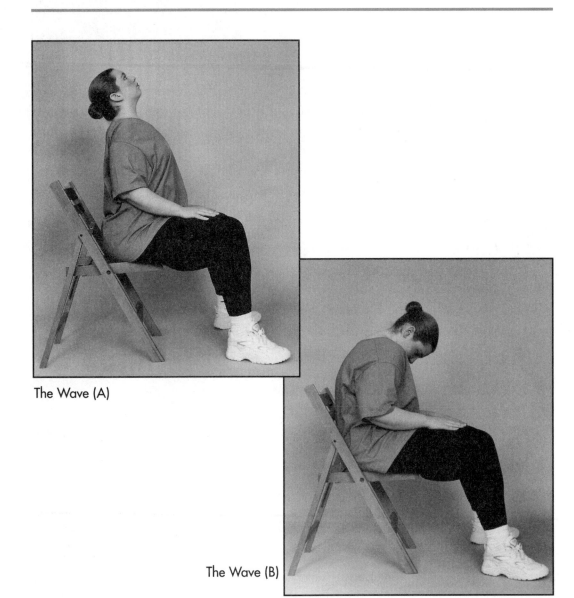

The Wave (A)

The Wave (B)

Technique Moment

The Wave stretches and massages the back and aids in spinal flexibility. It will assist in keeping the spine in optimal condition.

8. BALL SQUEEZE (ADDUCTORS/INNER THIGHS)

Start Position

Sit on a chair with the ball between your thighs. The ball should be as close to your pelvis as possible. Feet are parallel and chair width apart.

The Exercise

1. Inhale.
2. As you exhale, squeeze the ball and pull in your abdominals at the same time.
3. Inhale and release.
4. Repeat 12 times.

Technique Moment

To increase the intensity, try bringing your feet closer together, then squeeze the ball.

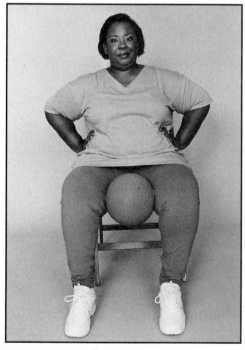

Ball Squeeze (A)

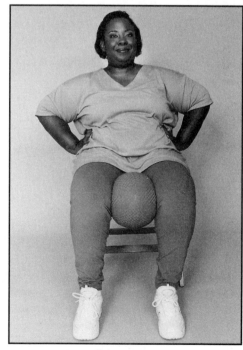

Ball Squeeze (B)

9. ABS ON THE INCLINE (ABDOMINALS)

Start Position

If you are using a STEP, set it up with three blocks on one end and one block on the other end. Lying on the incline, place the ball between your thighs, closer to your pelvis. Hands are clasped lightly behind the head.

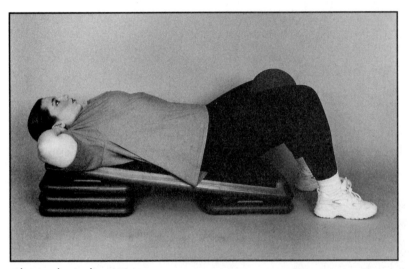

Abs on the Incline (A)

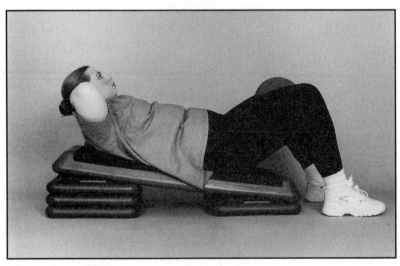

Abs on the Incline (B)

The Exercise
1. Inhale.

2. As you exhale, lift upward, bringing the rib cage toward the hips instead of lifting your head. You should feel the muscles in the upper part of the abdomen working.

3. Inhale and lower.

4. Repeat 12 times.

Technique Moment
Proper technique means using the hands to support the weight of the head and not using them to hoist the body up. Hands can also go over the abdominals to feel them working. The incline is meant to assist you (by means of gravity) to maximize use of the abdominals. Remember to maximize your Breathing for Me technique by bringing the navel to the spine as you lift up. This exercise can also be performed in a recliner chair.

SECTION IV: MEDITATION

Today's meditation is focused on breath and personal power. Change the music to something softer and close your eyes and follow your breath. Notice as you inhale that the belly rises, and as you exhale the belly falls. Now notice the space between your individual breaths—the brief moment of stillness at the end of an exhalation and before the next inhalation. In these brief moments, become aware of feelings of peace and personal power. You no longer have to look for external remedies to comfort and soothe you—it is right here, between the breaths. It may be difficult at first to sit quietly in this stillness. But once you become aware of it, returning to it is like wrapping a warm, soft terry cloth robe around you.

WEEK THREE: HELLO HAMSTRINGS
Theme for the Week: Connect (To Your Body and to the Earth)

Goals:

1. Complete 15 minutes of movement, even if this means walking in place.

2. Begin to understand the connection between breath and muscles, and how they affect your activities of daily living.

Exercises:

Section I ✦ Warm-up

Section II ✦ Your Personal Aerobic Program—Third 5 Minutes

Section III ✦ Strength Training and Stretching Techniques

    10. Modified Squats

    11. Hamstrings

    12. Adductors/Inner Thigh

    13. Leg Lift

Equipment:

1. Mat for floor (optional)
2. Chair
3. Pillow
4. Music
5. Water

SECTION I: WARM-UP

Keep in mind, the Warm-up (Section I) remains the same for the six-week program. If necessary, return to Week 1 to refresh your memory.

SECTION II: YOUR PERSONAL AEROBIC PROGRAM—THIRD 5 MINUTES

Add a third piece of music today for the Third 5 Minutes. You might try a song by Aretha Franklin or Tina Turner. Play your two other songs first, building on the choreography you have previously learned, and then add in your third piece with the following new moves. (I recommend taping your sequential music on a cassette so that it becomes your personalized workout routine. This way, if you travel a lot, you can take it with you. Just think of all the women of size across the country with their personalized power music jammin' toward fitness!) Here are a few more suggestions for added moves to your routine:

Arabesque is a term I borrow from the dance world. Step forward on your right leg, reaching your arms forward. Reach the left leg back as high as you can. Rock back on the left foot. Repeat the Arabesque 12 times, then change so that you begin with the left foot forward first. You might feel your hamstrings (back of the thighs) tighten immediately. Keep moving unless the muscles tighten painfully. If that is the case, stop, put your leg up on an ottoman or chair, and allow the back of the thigh to stretch out gently.

The Washing Machine move is a great one to help with something called internal rotation, or the ability to turn the legs in the hip sockets. Therefore, in this exercise, the navel always faces front as the knee comes across the torso. Most women tend to walk with their feet turned out, so this move helps to counteract the imbalance. It's fun and cute! Turn in your right foot and knee and touch your foot in front of you. Now the left. Your arms should swish away from the turned-in foot (when turning in on the right foot, your arms should swish to the right). Continue for a set of 8 and then do it while lifting the knees up and across, with that same washing machine feeling.

Technique Moment

Use your abdominals and don't overturn your feet, which could cause pain in the knees. Be sure to work the rotation from the hips.

SECTION III: STRENGTH TRAINING AND STRETCHING TECHNIQUES

10. MODIFIED SQUATS (QUADRICEPS AND GLUTEALS)

Start Position

Begin in a standing position approximately 8 inches from the chair and facing away from the chair. Feet are hip-width apart, toes pointing straight ahead.

The Exercise

1. Bend your legs and reach your tailbone back (stick your butt out!). While this move is not "dainty," it will assure proper technique for your program.

2. Continue bending forward, reaching your tailbone back and bending the legs until you end up seated on the chair.

3. Rest.

4. Inhale. Then, as you exhale, come up from the chair, pushing your legs into the earth like strong tree trunks. Keep your hands on your thighs.

5. Repeat the sequence 8 to 12 times.

Technique Moment

You should feel this exercise in the top of the thighs and buttocks. You should not feel this in the knees. If you do, try taking your buttocks further back, and

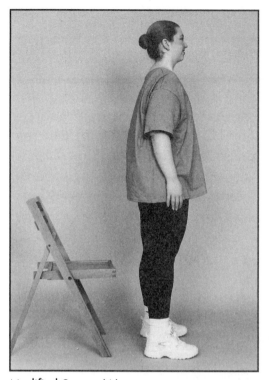

Modified Squats (A)

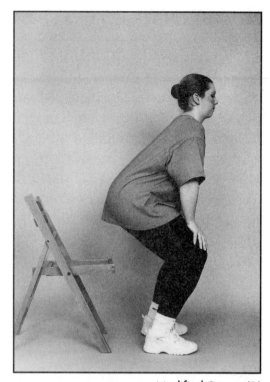

Modified Squats (B)

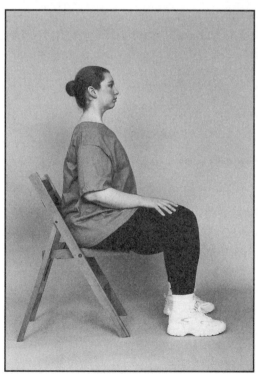

Modified Squats (C)

be sure to counterbalance by bringing the torso forward at a 45-degree angle. You can also have someone assist you in the beginning to ensure proper technique. Use your hands to push on your thighs. Your hands can help control the descent and assist you in rising to a standing position. This is the introduction to proper technique for squats. If, with time, the exercise starts to get easy, remove the chair and squat, using the image of a public toilet as your guide. This is an excellent exercise with regard to activities of daily living and functional fitness (up and down from chairs, sofas, and toilets).

11. HAMSTRINGS

Start Position

Lie on your stomach with the pillow under your lower stomach and hips to support your lower back. If you cannot get down to the floor, this exercise can also be done on your bed until you feel more comfortable.

The Exercise

1. Curl the right foot under.
2. Bend your left leg at a right angle, with the sole of the foot facing the ceiling.
3. Inhale.
4. As you exhale, push the foot up to the ceiling bringing the navel to the spine.
5. Inhale and lower the knee to the floor.
6. Exhale and push the foot up again.
7. Repeat 8 to 12 times and then change legs.

Technique Moment

You should feel this exercise in the hamstrings (back of the thigh) of the lifting leg as well as in the buttocks. If your lower back hurts, try readjusting the pillow, pulling the abs in more as you lift. You can also modify this exercise by not lifting the leg so high. A second modification: In a standing position, place your foot up against a surface such as a door frame. Push and release 12 times.

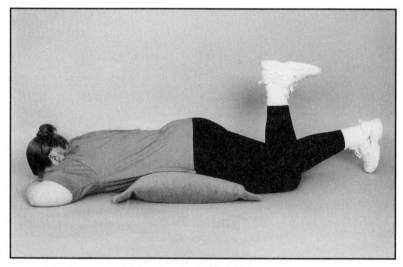

Hamstrings (A)

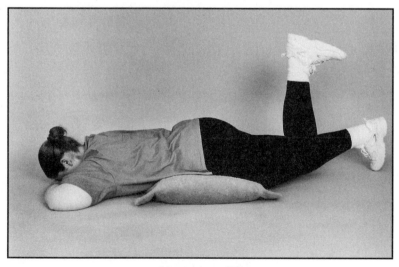

Hamstrings (B)

12. INNER THIGH (ADDUCTORS)

Start Position

Lie down on your right side. Bend the left leg and tuck a pillow underneath it for support.

The Exercise

1. Stretch the right arm and right leg out straight.
2. Inhale.

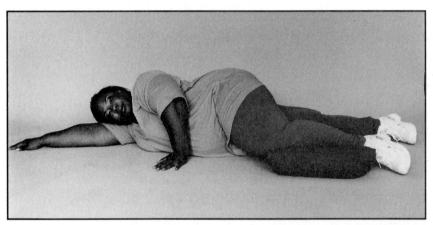

Inner Thigh (A)

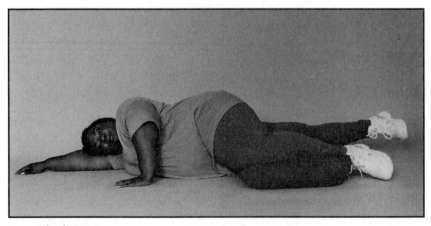

Inner Thigh (B)

3. As you exhale, bring the right leg straight up to the ceiling, elongating the spine.

4. Inhale as you lower the leg.

5. Repeat 8 to 12 times.

6. Change to the other side by rolling onto your back.

Technique Moment

In this exercise we are trying to access the inner thigh muscles, which run from the pubic bone down the inside of the thigh to the knee area. These mus-

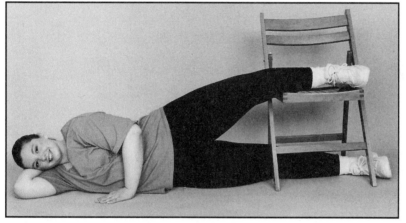

Inner Thigh Variation (A)

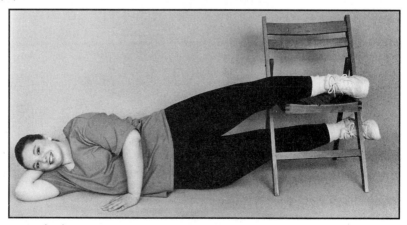

Inner Thigh Variation (B)

cles tend to be weak in women—perhaps because of leg width and/or our naturally wider pelvis. Take your time with this exercise, and be certain to maintain proper technique. A variation would be putting the left leg up on a chair and lengthening the right leg underneath as seen in the photos. Lift and lower the lower leg 12 times and repeat on the other side. If you cannot go to the floor, a third variation for accessing the inner thigh muscles would begin by standing in a wide parallel. In your mind, draw your feet together (as if you were ice skating) without actually moving the feet. You should feel a slight tension on the inner thigh muscles.

13. LEG LIFTS (QUADRICEPS, HIP FLEXORS)

Start Position
Lying on your back, bend the left knee until the foot rests on the floor and extend the right leg out straight.

The Exercise
1. Inhale.
2. As you exhale, engage your abdominals and lift the right leg up until it is parallel with the left knee (a 45-degree angle).
3. Inhale as you lower the leg to the calf height of the left leg.
4. Repeat 8 to 12 times and then change sides.

Technique Moment
Be careful not to spill out (no abdominal support) as you lower the leg. Try to maintain the neutral position of the spine by using the abdominals. To change the focus of the exercise, try lowering the leg for a count of ten, keeping the abdominal wall strong. You may feel the back of the thigh (hamstrings) working.

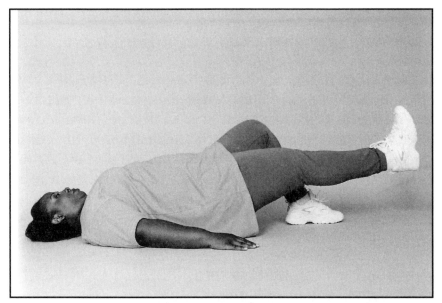

Leg Lifts (A)

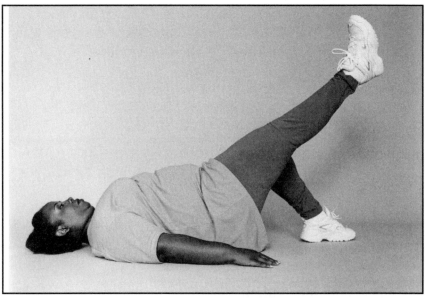

Leg Lifts (B)

SECTION IV: MEDITATION

Put on soft music. As you sit in a chair or lie down on your back, close your eyes and focus on your breath. As you sink deeper into relaxation, picture a tiny seed buried in the Earth. As the seed starts to grow, its roots extend downward. The roots are the anchor for a tree that will stand tall and proud, much as your legs will secure you as you walk with a heightened posture. As the limbs of the tree continue to grow upward toward the sun, so does your body revel in the beauty of its newfound strength—your connection to your muscles and the Earth.

WEEK FOUR: STEPPING OUT
Theme for the Week: All Movement Is Great!

Goals:
1. Complete 20 minutes of movement, even if it means walking in place.
2. Feel more power through the arms and chest.
3. Experience strength and length in the lower leg.

Exercises:
Section I ✦ Warm-up
Section II ✦ Your Personal Aerobic Program—Last 5 Minutes
Section III ✦ Strength Training and Stretching Techniques
    14. Titanic
    15. Wall Push-up
    16. Calf Stretch, Calf Raise, Toe Tap
    17. Cobra

Section IV ✦ Meditation

Equipment:
1. Mat for the floor (optional)
2. Chair
3. Stairs or telephone book
4. Music
5. Water

SECTION I AND SECTION II: WARM-UP AND YOUR PERSONAL AEROBIC PROGRAM—LAST 5 MINUTES

Follow Warm-up from Weeks 1 to 3. By Week 4, you are now ready to complete 20 minutes of continuous movement, rather than just 5 minutes. You may have started a walking program with a friend, or perhaps you are ready to choose a piece of music as your grand finale for Weeks 4 through 6. Try something powerful and strong like the theme from *Rocky* or Gloria Gaynor's "I Will Survive." Connect all your choreography from the previous 3 weeks and add the following to your routine:

If you choose the theme from *Rocky*, I recommend our Sports Move sequence: Stepping forward on the left foot, bowl with your right hand and then rock back on the right foot. Repeat the bowling motion 8 times, and then switch to a tennis serve. Toss the ball up from the left hand and serve with the right making a big sweeping motion with your imaginary racket. You can then move on to golf swings, dribbling a basketball, swinging a bat, and playing volleyball. If you decide to work with some music like "I Will Survive," choose more of a show-girl approach. We enjoy mimicking the Rockettes by holding out our arms and kicking our legs straight ahead. We also enjoy doing *Soul Train* or the stroll—pretend you are dancing down between two lines of people on either side of you. You can do either the pony, the hustle, or whatever makes you feel good. Just be sure to keep moving. Sing along to the music if you wish, and be sure to take a grand bow at the end! Congratulations on completing 20 minutes of movement!

SECTION III: STRENGTH TRAINING AND STRETCHING TECHNIQUES

14. TITANIC

This is one of my favorites. Because we tend to stand with rounded shoulders, this exercise helps open up the chest and enhance your posture.

The Exercise

1. Stand with your left foot slightly in front of the right—not in a straight line, but slightly apart.

2. Roll your shoulders back and reach both arms back behind you with palms facing in.

3. Reach and release the arms 8 times, bringing the shoulder blades together.

4. Change legs and repeat.

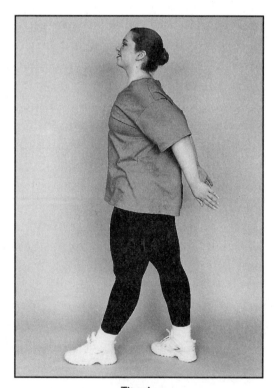

Titanic

Technique Moment

Imagine you are Kate Winslet, standing on the bow of the *Titanic* with Leo by your side. Feel your chest muscles stretch and your lungs expand as you let in the bracing sea air. Look up slightly as though feeling the sun on your face, while your arms stretch behind you.

15. WALL PUSH-UP

Start Position

Place both hands on the wall, about shoulder-width apart. Elbows should be in line with the shoulders.

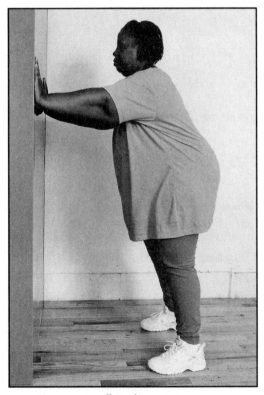
Wall Push-up (A)

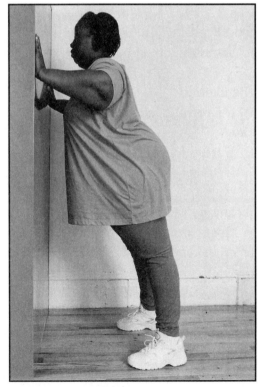
Wall Push-up (B)

The Exercise

1. Inhale as you bend the elbows, bringing the chest closer to the wall.

2. As you exhale, push away from the wall, straightening the elbows and returning to start position.

3. Repeat 8 times.

Technique Moment

Be sure to keep your body in one long line, from your heels through the crown of your head. Don't arch your back. Send your heels into the floor as you reach your head upward toward the ceiling.

16. CALF STRETCH, CALF RAISE, TOE TAP

Start Position

Stand on a telephone book or the bottom step of the stairs.

The Exercise

1. Drop the left heel off the back of the step until you feel the stretch in the calf.

2. Hold for 30 seconds.

3. Repeat on the right.

Technique Moment

Most women experience tight calves from carrying the body forward in their feet in order to balance their bodies. Take your time with this stretch and be certain not to lock the knee of the back foot. You can also add Calf Raises as shown. Rise up and down on the toes 12 times. For the second set, bend the knees as you lower down (heels should be on the floor). Pretend you are shooting a basketball without actually jumping off the floor.

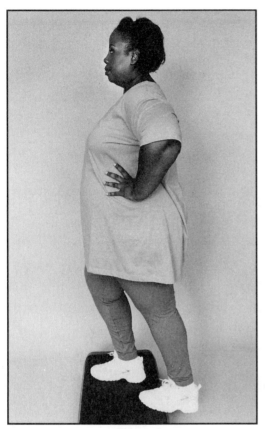

Calf Stretch

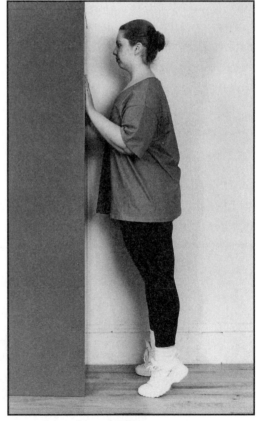

Calf Raise

Toe taps can also be incorporated to complete a total lower leg conditioning program.

Start Position

Sit on a chair with your feet straight out in front of you.

The Exercise

1. Lift your left toes off the floor, pulling up from the front of the shin.
2. Repeat on the right foot.
3. Continue alternating the feet as if pumping the gas pedal of a car. Continue the exercise for about one minute.

Technique Moment

You should feel a dull ache in the front of the shins. This is where people experience shin splints—a painful condition in the shins. Strengthening this muscle will help guard against shin splints and assist with agility and overall balance.

17. COBRA

Start Position

Lie on your stomach with your palms down near your shoulders. If you cannot get to the floor, try the exercise on your bed.

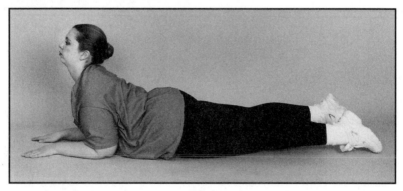

Cobra

The Exercise

1. Inhale.
2. As you exhale, slowly lift your chest by pressing into your palms. Actively reach your chest forward.
3. Inhale as you lower.
4. Repeat 4 to 8 times.

Technique Moment

If there is lower back discomfort, try bringing the navel toward the spine and reaching the chest more forward. If there is still discomfort, do not come up as high. If you experience sharp shooting pain, do not continue.

SECTION IV: MEDITATION

With soft music, close your eyes and focus on your breath. As you begin to relax, think of an animal that is representative of you. It could be a bird, a cat, or a tiger. Notice how easily this animal moves through its surroundings, stretching naturally and running or flying freely. Picture yourself as that animal and feel how your body moves freely through space, without aches and pains or interference. All movement is great, and you are entitled to a life of movement. Proceed through your week with the strength, confidence, and assurance of the animal that moves freely within you.

WEEK FIVE: PUTTING IT ALL TOGETHER
Theme for the Week: The Flow of Movement

Goals:

1. Maintain 20 minutes of movement.
2. Increase your range of exercises by performing larger movements.

Exercises:

Section I ✦ Warm-up

Section II ✦ Your Personal Aerobic Program—20 Minutes of Movement

Section III ✦ Strength Training and Stretching Techniques

      18. Seated Quad Strength

      19. Rowing Machine

      20. Cat Stretch

      21. Wall Slide

Section IV ✦ Meditation

Equipment:

1. Mat for the floor (optional)
2. Chair
3. STEP (optional) or bed
4. Towel
5. Dynaband (optional) or towel
6. Music
7. Water

SECTION I AND SECTION II: WARM-UP AND YOUR PERSONAL AEROBIC PROGRAM—20 MINUTES OF MOVEMENT

Begin with your Warm-up (Week 1) and then pop in your tape of your four motivating songs and begin your 20 minutes of aerobic movement (Week 4). Your body should already be very familiar with the movement, and if new moves come to you during your songs, try them out! Movement is all about the freedom of the soul—let your spirit shine as you move freely about the house. If your songs no longer inspire you, change them! This is the base of your routine, so make sure it puts you in an energetic mood that will pump you up with energy and enthusiasm! I have also provided a list of music companies in the Resources section of this manual. You may find some of them helpful in your program.

SECTION III: STRENGTH TRAINING AND STRETCHING TECHNIQUES

18. SEATED QUAD STRENGTH

Start Position

Sit on the STEP or on your bed with the right leg extended forward and the left leg hanging down to the floor. Tuck a towel under the right knee.

The Exercise

1. Keeping your heel down on the STEP or bed, press the back of the knee into the towel. Watch as the kneecap (patella) slides horizontally toward your torso as the thigh muscles (quadriceps) contract. Hold for a count of 5 and release.

2. Repeat 4 to 8 times.

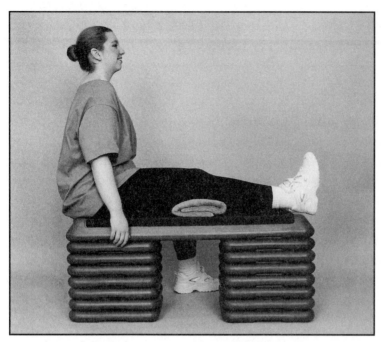

Seated Quad Strength

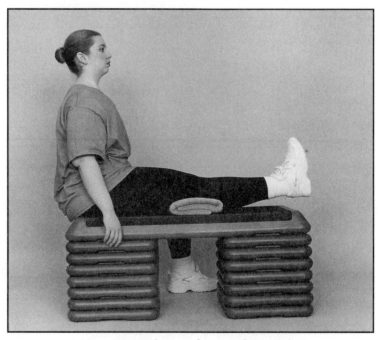

Improper Technique for Quad Strength

Technique Moment

This exercise is extremely difficult and may cause your thigh muscles to cramp up. Keep in mind this exercise is intended to strengthen the thigh muscles so that you use them, and not your knees, to help support your body. The second photo shows improper technique, or How *Not* to Do This Exercise. The knee is incorrectly locked and bowing the leg. This is called hyperextension. If you adopt this hyperextended position, the front of the leg (quadriceps) is not working and the back of the leg (hamstrings) is being overstretched.

19. ROWING MACHINE (RHOMBOIDS)

Start Position

Sit at the end of the STEP or bed or chair.

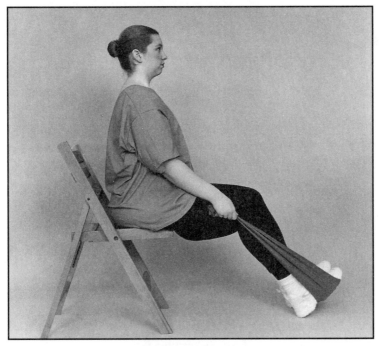

Rowing Machine (A)

The Exercise

1. Wrap the Dynaband around your arches.

2. Inhale.

3. As you exhale, gently pull the elbows back by your sides as if you were rowing a boat.

4. The shoulder blades will come together.

5. Hold for a moment and return to start position.

6. Repeat 12 times.

Technique Moment

This exercise will strengthen your posture and back muscles, and help some women carry a larger bust. The exercise should feel "busty." Sit tall, reach the spine long, and maintain that posture throughout the exercise with only the shoulder blades moving. The Dynaband adds resistance, but the exercise can be performed without it or with 1- to 3-pound free weights.

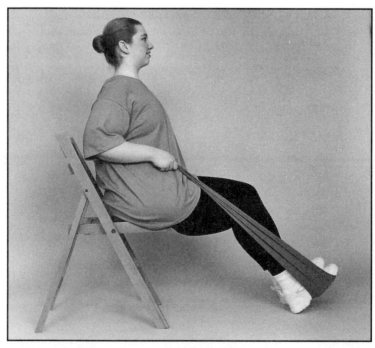

Rowing Machine (B)

20. CAT STRETCH

Start Position

Using a sturdy chair, place both hands on the chair seat.

The Exercise

1. Inhale, lifting the chin to the ceiling.
2. As you exhale, tuck the chin in to the chest and round the back like a cat.
3. Repeat 4 times and rest.

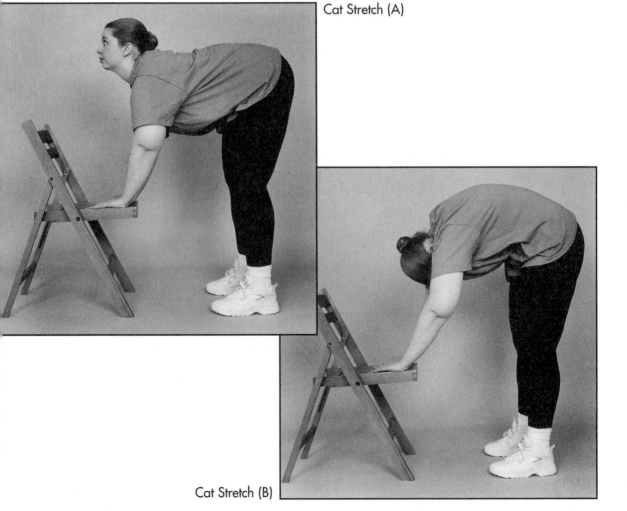

Cat Stretch (A)

Cat Stretch (B)

Technique Moment

Keep the knees soft at all times. Feet are hip-width apart. When you round your back like a cat, you should feel a stretch across the lower back. Feel the whole spine as a long curve, from the base of the skull to the tip of the tailbone. Every vertebra is participating in the movement.

21. WALL SLIDE

Start Position

Stand with your back against the wall, the feet about 8 inches from the wall.

The Exercise

1. Inhale.

2. As you exhale, slowly slide down the wall until you feel like you are sitting in a chair.

3. Hold for 4 counts.

4. Inhale.

5. Return to start position by pushing the feet into the floor and sliding to a standing position.

6. Repeat 4 to 8 times.

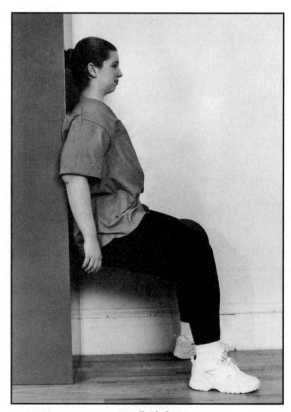

Wall Slide

Technique Moment

You can use the ball between the thighs for more stability and/or intensity. There should be no pain in the knees. If there is, do not slide so deeply. Buttocks should not slide lower than the knees, which should be parallel. Pretend you are sitting in an imaginary chair. While in the seated position of this exercise, try to keep your abdominals in and your shoulders and back of your head against the wall. To increase intensity, hold your arms out to your sides.

SECTION IV: MEDITATION

Close your eyes and settle into your breath. Imagine a river running freely, with no dams or obstacles to impede its progress. Now imagine the energy inside your body as a flowing river, and how it too can flow freely . . . without being impeded by aches and pains. The barriers have been broken and your body is able to move forward in life with grace and ease.

WEEK SIX: GRADUATION
Theme for the Week: I Am Beautiful Inside and Outside

Goals:
1. Understand the stretches and feel their importance.
2. Feel that the 20 minutes of movement is easier to accomplish.

Exercises:
Section I ✦ Warm-up
Section II ✦ Your Personal Aerobic Program—20 Minutes of Movement
Section III ✦ Strength Training and Stretching Techniques
     22. Shoulder Strength
     23. Neck Stretch
     24. Psoas Stretch
     25. Hamstring Stretch
Section IV ✦ Meditation

Equipment:
1. Mat for the floor (optional)
2. Towel
3. Chair
4. STEP (optional) or bed
5. Dynaband (optional)
6. Music
7. Water

SECTION I AND SECTION II: WARM-UP AND YOUR PERSONAL AEROBIC PROGRAM—20 MINUTES OF MOVEMENT

At the studio, we make the sixth session a grand affair. Many women have never been able to keep to a fitness commitment for a period of time. The fact that you have completed the six weeks proves to me that you have laid the foundation for an active lifestyle. By now, your empowering and motivating music is like a familiar friend. Pop in the tape or play that CD, and you are whisked away to an alternate universe where you can move freely. Begin with the standard Warm-up and segue into your 20 minutes of movement from the previous weeks.

SECTION III: STRENGTH TRAINING AND STRETCHING TECHNIQUES

We will complete the program with one shoulder-straightening exercise and then focus on the stretches most important for women of size. Once you have learned them, you can incorporate them throughout your program.

22. SHOULDER STRENGTH (ROTATOR CUFF)

Start Position

Hold your arms out to your sides like the letter T. Make fists with your hands, palms facing the floor.

The Exercise

1. Inhale.

2. As you exhale, draw small circles in a backward direction with the arms 12 times.

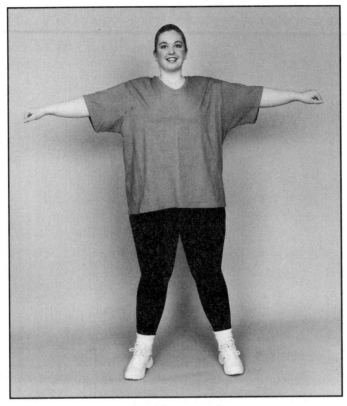

Shoulder Strength

3. Reverse the direction of the circles 12 times.

4. Depending on the strength of your shoulders, you can repeat the entire exercise until you feel a dull ache in the shoulder area.

Technique Moment

If there is any discomfort, try lowering the arms slightly. If there is still a problem, consult your doctor.

23. NECK STRETCH

Start Position

Sit on a chair looking straight ahead. Roll up a towel and place it behind your neck, holding it with both hands.

The Exercise

1. Inhale.
2. As you exhale, gently stretch your chin toward the ceiling, eyes looking upward.
3. Inhale and return to center.
4. Repeat 4 times.

Technique Moment

As you return your head to the center, you may feel a bit light-headed. This

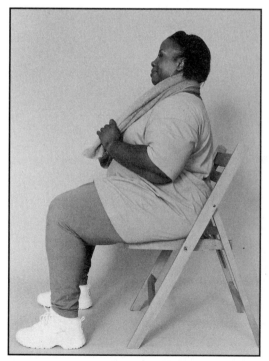 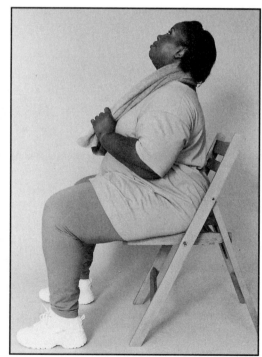

Neck Stretch (A)   Neck Stretch (B)

response is normal and should decrease as your range of motion improves and proper alignment is enhanced.

24. PSOAS STRETCH

Start Position

Lie on your back on the STEP or bed with your legs bent and feet resting on the surface.

The Exercise

1. Bring your left knee to your chest.
2. Wrap a towel or Dynaband behind your left thigh.
3. Inhale.
4. As you exhale, slowly lower your right leg off the bench or bed until you feel a stretch on the top of the right thigh, deep in the hip.
5. Inhale.

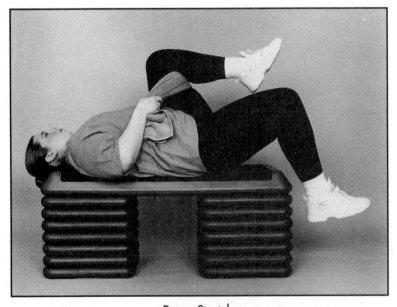

Psoas Stretch

6. As you exhale, bring the right leg back in toward your chest and return to start position.

7. Repeat on the other side.

Technique Moment

This is a very strong stretch for the psoas, a muscle that runs across the hip to the lower back. Use strong abdominals and be sure not to arch your back as you lower the leg.

25. HAMSTRING STRETCH

Start Position

Lie on your back and place the towel or Dynaband around your right foot. Keep the left leg bent on the floor.

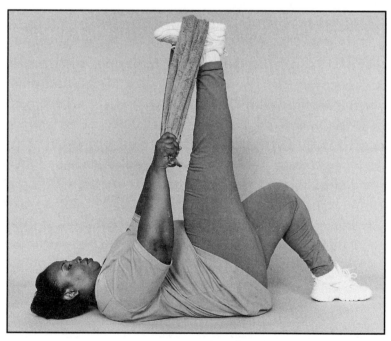

Hamstring Stretch

The Exercise

1. Inhale.
2. As you exhale, stretch your right leg up to the ceiling.
3. Inhale.
4. As you exhale, gently stretch your thigh closer to your chest keeping your leg straight but not locked.
5. Flex your foot, bringing your toes toward your nose.
6. Repeat the inhale and exhale 4 times.
7. Change sides.

Technique Moment

You should feel the first part of this stretch on the back of your thigh. When you flex the foot, you should feel the stretch in the calf muscle. Stretch gently.

SECTION IV: MEDITATION

Change the music and notice your breath, using the same technique as we have all along. Focus on the rise and fall of your breath and then notice the space between the breaths. In this relaxed state, honor your body as sacred and precious, deserving of delicate care and safety. Imagine all the precious gifts you'd like to give to your body: brisk walks out-of-doors, sunlight, fresh air, the sensation of cool, refreshing breezes on skin. Thank your body for carrying you through life and allowing you the opportunity for this incredible journey.

This program has prepared you structurally to be able to participate in numerous activities without pain or injury. Most people think of physical fitness as a chore and a bore, akin to "doing time." But this program has prepared you for other activities such as bowling or joining a yoga class, or even trying a fitness activity from your youth. Perhaps you once liked ballroom dancing. Or have harbored a secret desire to learn how to play tennis. Once you've finished the six-week course, your next goal is to begin to take part in life in a way you were previously afraid or unable to do. You can even partner up with friends and help to motivate each other. This program is the link from an inactive lifestyle to one filled with joy and movement.

You may wish to start the program again, in order to ensure that exercise becomes a habit. Some women come to my studio for the introductory course and repeat it in order to develop a high level of confidence. I recommend you make the commitment to maintaining a movement program in your life, and incorporate elements from this program. You will be pleasantly surprised by how many movements and techniques your body "remembers" as you venture out into new fitness endeavors.

CHAPTER EIGHT

MAINTAINING AN ACTIVE LIFESTYLE

We are what we repeatedly do.
Excellence, therefore, is not an act, but a habit.
—Aristotle

It's a guarantee—movement will make you feel better. The moment you set your body in motion your blood starts flowing, your oxygen intake increases, your muscles start pumping—and your mood is lifted, your health improved, your energy fortified. Changing your physiology by moving provides that "quick fix" we are all looking for, a source of immediate gratification. However, even though movement feels so terrific, sometimes it's difficult to work fitness into our lives. A myriad of demands on our time seem to get in the way. Instead of judging yourself harshly, keep these points in mind:

1. Fitness is not an all-or-nothing proposition. You don't have to adhere to a fitness routine worthy of an Army Basic Training recruit to be fit. Any amount of movement that you can incorporate into your lifestyle beats a standing date with the TV.

2. Focus on increasing your activities of daily living, such as picking up your children, carrying groceries, even climbing stairs instead of taking the elevator. These, rather than numbers on a scale, are the measurements of your success.

3. Remember that fitness creates a ripple effect on other women around you: daughters, mother, sisters, mentors, colleagues, friends. Through your example, you empower others to move. I truly believe that the actions of an individual

affect the collective consciousness of all people. Therefore, your commitment to movement contributes to a shift in the consciousness of those around you.

In this journey, there will be setbacks along the way. I would be lying if I said otherwise. Many women feel "life" gets in the way of prioritizing their health. Factors include:

✦ Career promotion
✦ Death of a loved one
✦ Divorce
✦ Family stress
✦ Illness
✦ Injury
✦ Job stress
✦ Marriage
✦ New baby
✦ Relationship troubles
✦ Weather

Yes, even good things can get in the way. Some of us make improvements in our lives, then begin to feel we are not worthy of those improvements. So we self-sabotage; for every step forward, we seem determined to take two steps back. Sometimes even feeling good can kick up fears: fears of the unknown, fear of change, fear of success. It may seem easier to go back to what is familiar rather than blaze new trails. You may get overwhelmed and discouraged, spinning you back into the vicious cycle of hopelessness and inactivity.

When a setback occurs, keep these points in mind:

1. Think of exercise as akin to learning how to ride a bicycle. If you've fallen, dust yourself off and try again! Similarly, if you've gotten out of the habit of moving, don't beat yourself up. Instead, read one of the real women's stories of inspiration that I've included in the Appendix to help keep you going. They are sure to inspire you to stick with the program.

2. Don't judge yourself. If you feel as though you have failed, ask yourself this: By whose standards am I failing? The very question motivates one to reexamine old internal rules and judgments.

3. You are not alone. Many women have felt the same way you do right now. If you're having trouble motivating yourself on your own behalf, imagine that you're doing it so that other women can draw from your strength.

4. Successful people usually "fail" many times before they succeed. Babe Ruth struck out numerous times before he hit his first home run. Albert Einstein was a miserable student. Critics denounced Van Gogh's works. The key to success is the ability to hold on to your goals and persevere through the ups and downs.

5. You are worthy. Remember that fitness makes room in your soul for feelings of self-worth, as you begin to see yourself as capable and powerful.

This book is only a beginning. As you become more accustomed to movement and fitness, you will feel more comfortable in traditional gyms, exercise classes, and situations where you will mix with people of all sizes and body types. As your comfort level increases you may wish to:

1. Try out a gym, and share your knowledge about this program with a trainer.

2. Connect with other like-minded women in your neighborhood and form fitness groups.

3. Try fitness activities you haven't attempted since you were a child, such as ice skating and swimming.

4. Organize or participate in fitness activities in your workplace or community such as bowling parties, walkathons, and dances.

The only thing certain about life is change. Therefore it is important to maintain a balance with all your various activities: work-related, familial, social, personal, and fitness-related. However, fitness should not be relegated to last on the list. It provides a base for all the other activities, and a place for you to reconnect with yourself when life starts to become too hectic. Fitness is where you regain balance.

CHAPTER NINE

FOOD FOR THOUGHT

Insanity is doing the same thing over and over again,
but expecting different results.
—Rita Mae Brown

Food is an issue at the center of many women's lives. It often creates anxiety, and you may have developed a dysfunctional relationship to food. Since my work is devoted to women of size, what I realize is that I am in the company of extraordinary experts on dieting. Most of you can make lists of foods deemed "acceptable" and "unacceptable" by the diet industry, and count calories and fat grams with the skill of high-level medical researchers. You've tried every dieting technique: fasting and food combining, liquid protein and meal substitutes, high-fat, low-fat, and seemingly no-fat regimens, hamburgers, grapefruit, and cabbage soup. And after years of dieting, you've discovered the simple truth: Diets don't work. In fact, with the rise of a multibillion-dollar diet industry and the proliferation of diet doctors and weight loss clinics, our nation is steadily getting heavier.

While the fact that diets fail may contradict everything you've ever been told about fitness and weight, it's a truth most women I've worked with have already discovered. It's important first to clarify our meaning of the word "diet." We use the term to signify a regimen that restricts food intake and/or labels some foods unacceptable. Some diets call for foods that are difficult to obtain or prepare for people on the go. Others are exceedingly limited and repetitive, dooming the dieter to a bland and joyless regimen. While many dieters lose weight in the short term, they rarely keep it off. Once the dieters return to their old eating habits, they gain back the weight, and often more. What's worse, repeat dieting can end up harming the body by confusing and even permanently altering the metabolism.

To get the full picture of why dieting is so pernicious, it's important to understand this last point: Your body is accustomed to utilizing a steady number of calories per day. Diets tend to restrict calories. While the body will respond in the short term by burning up stored energy in the form of fat (or, for extreme diets, lean muscle), over time its response changes. When faced with long-term caloric restrictions, the body begins to operate in "conservation mode," requiring fewer and fewer calories to get through the day. The metabolism actually begins to slow down. As a result, the woman who once maintained her weight at 2,400 calories a day may now only consume 2,000 calories a day for the same results.

Most people's metabolisms bounce back to pre-diet levels (adjusted to the new lower weight) after the diet is finished, but repeat dieting may alter the metabolism and slow it down permanently. Even after the diet is finished and the dieter begins to incorporate more calories into her daily intake, the metabolism is still prepared for a starvation scenario, and is operating at a snail's pace. When rich foods are reintroduced, the body no longer knows what to do with them. The result? Weight gain. Subsequent diets may become more and more extreme and restrictive, yet have less and less of an effect. Complicating matters further is the fact that over time a repeat dieter is getting older, so her body is naturally utilizing fewer calories as her metabolism slows down during each decade of adulthood. Dieting also sabotages a woman's efforts at weight loss. Each time a dieter goes on an extreme, restrictive diet, not only does she lose fat, but she also loses lean body mass in the form of muscle. Muscle is more metabolically active than fat and burns more calories, so when lean body mass is lost the metabolism slows. This is one reason why exercise is so important:

Strength training and exercise build muscle, which burns extra calories. Fitness is the key to a happy, healthy life.

Overall exercise raises the body's metabolic rate all day long. The woman who exercises utilizes more calories—not just while she's exercising, but throughout the day and even while she sleeps. It is for this reason that the program in *Real Fitness for Real Women* focuses on movement and exercise as a whole.

I believe that women of size don't need more reminders about the importance of eating well. I am so keenly aware of the myth that all large women are compulsive eaters or binge eaters. However, when it comes to food and eating there's something far more complex at work for many of us: our thoughts and feelings. Through my eating struggles, I have learned to recognize these thoughts and feelings as a complex and continuous internal dialogue, teaching me to pinpoint both my nutritional and emotional needs. I am constantly challenged by the idea of developing skills around food to assess my emotions. Now, instead of dieting or bingeing, as I have in the past, I ask myself four basic questions:

1. What do I *not* want to feel?
2. What do I *really* want or need right now? Is it company? Solitude? Comfort? Affirmation?
3. If it's truly hunger, I ask myself, "*What* do I want to eat?"
4. If it's emotional eating, I ask myself: "*What* can I do instead of eating that is *constructive rather than destructive?*"

These questions enabled me to stop my familiar response to food, and allowed me to set new patterns. If you are about to binge, ask yourself these questions. Think about the answers. Understand why you are eating and if you really want to.

When I started on this chapter I consulted with Barbara Gewirtz, M.S., R.D., a nutritionist and a former nutrition and fitness editor of *Good Housekeeping*. In addition to her work as a nutritionist, Barbara is a plus-size woman and a participant of the *Real Fitness for Real Women* program. She offers the insights of a woman who is fit, healthy, and proud of her strong, graceful body. Together,

Barbara and I have designed ways to help heal dysfunctional eating habits, as well as heal the metabolism. As I stated earlier, dieting often damages the metabolism and throws one's entire eating patterns out of whack.

But it is possible to correct your eating habits, and it is also possible to heal the metabolism from the damage wreaked by years of dieting. The food suggestions I recommend are tools for recovery that have helped me. To embark on these you have to be willing to reject all your current eating habits and everything you have ever heard about dieting, and replace them with a desire to eat well, pay attention to feelings of hunger and fullness, and learn to truly enjoy your meals.

The problem with any sort of compulsive eating, whether or not you're overeating, is that while you may be focused on the food itself, as you eat you aren't really in touch with your body. When you can reverse that—when you are in touch with your body—you know what you want and need, you know when to begin, and you know when to stop. The following list of suggestions for healthier eating can help you gently modify your eating—and living—habits in order to maximize your health. Take these lifestyle suggestions one at a time. Do not try for enormous changes all at once or go overboard. Gradual change is the key to success.

1. DON'T CALL IT A DIET

To reiterate: You need to remove the word "diet" from your vocabulary! The word "diet" is inextricably linked in our minds with deprivation. One can almost see the Food Police coming to your kitchen and emptying the fridge. A diet is meant to be temporary—for every diet, there is an equal and opposite binge. I know it's scary to give up the notion of dieting when not being on one usually leads to thoughts of self-destructive behavior. But diets encourage women to think of food in terms of good and bad. And all-or-nothing thinking is responsible for so much of our society's dysfunctional relationship to food.

Do not deprive yourself of your favorite foods. Diversity is important. You should simply create an eating lifestyle that works for you. The goal, in place of yet another diet, is to eat a wide variety of foods that are nutritious, tasty, and celebratory as a natural and joyful extension of living.

2. HEED YOUR HUNGER

For many of you, eating has been so fraught with tension and guilt that you've learned to distrust your feelings of fullness and hunger. But that trust can also be relearned. Relearning what hunger and satiation feel like are essential to this program.

As you start to exercise, you begin to notice more distinctive feelings of hunger and thirst. Pay attention, and answer those internal needs with healthy choices. Your body speaks to you loudly and clearly: Listen carefully! Your body is a smarter, more complex, and more sophisticated organism than anything ever created by man; it knows what it needs, and it will give you that information if you just tune in.

Many of you, unaware of the sensation of hunger, are accustomed to eating past the point of fullness. Since many of you have learned to eat to fulfill emotional needs, not just physical ones, no amount of food ever really seems like enough. You must learn to put food and eating back in their proper perspective—to learn when you're hungry and when you're sated. Give yourself enough time between meals so that hunger whispers quietly in your ear—but not so much time that it screams like a mad banshee!

3. SATISFY YOUR CRAVINGS

Of course, when some of us tune in, all we hear is, "Give me chocolate!" Again, listen to your body! If your body says, "Chocolate, and only chocolate will do," chances are a few squares of the finest, richest chocolate will satisfy your sweet tooth (whereas twenty Hershey Bars will definitely be overkill!). You should incorporate that moderate amount into your eating habits. After all, food is for enjoyment as well as nutrition, and you may in fact have a psychological need for chocolate every now and again (who doesn't?).

How you answer those cravings is important. You must learn to enjoy "forbidden foods" in moderation. I know this may sound counterintuitive, but it's important to eat foods that you've been told, or you have told yourself, that you shouldn't. If chocolate is what you crave, you can incorporate the taste as a low-fat pudding every day. That way the taste of chocolate won't necessarily precipitate a binge. Remember: There are no good and bad foods, just good and bad food habits.

When you deny yourself certain foods, you lose the ability to eat them sensibly. Let me offer as an example the case of apple pie. Let's say you've internalized the idea of apple pie as a "bad" food. You try to avoid it, but can't, because like small children most of us secretly want what we have been denied. So inevitably, in a moment of "weakness," you reach for the pie that you crave. Then, feeling as though you've already been "bad," you overindulge and eat past the point where you're actually enjoying the taste.

Since no food, not even fresh apple pie, signifies personal weakness, why shouldn't you be able to enjoy this pleasure in moderation? Instead of eating your apple pie in the house, have it in a restaurant. Sit down, order the pie, then really savor it. Eat it slowly, bit by bit, until that last bit of crust is finished. Feel the sensation of satisfying fullness, and thank yourself for this delicious treat. Eating slowly will enhance your eating awareness and allow you to more fully savor your food.

4. EAT SITTING DOWN

Eat while you're sitting down—preferably at a dining table, and not sprawled on the sofa in front of the TV. Similarly, although many of us enjoy talking on the phone while we eat, it is better to eat with someone face-to-face or eat without distraction. It's difficult to develop healthful eating habits when the mind is not focused clearly on the food in front of you. When it is, however, you have a chance to truly enjoy what you are eating, as well as focus on how your body feels as you eat it.

5. REFUEL REGULARLY

Plan snacks between meals so you never reach the point of sharp, gnawing hunger. Start by planning three meals, or alternatively four smaller meals, each day, and allow yourself healthy snacks such as fruit or carrot sticks in between. (Low-fat puddings, popcorn, or string cheese are also great snacks.) Make sure to eat at regular intervals, not going for more than three or four hours at a time without food.

Eating at regular intervals is the first step to monitoring your body's cues. Throughout the day you will feel both mildly hungry and full, and with time this range becomes more familiar. As these sensations become clearer, you may end up eating more or less than you had planned. For example, you may plan to eat half a sandwich for lunch, and find that half a sandwich suffices. Or you may opt for two pieces of chicken instead of one with dinner as your body tells you that it needs the extra protein and calories. Eating to the point of satisfaction, and not before or beyond, will heal your body and bring you to your optimal weight. Your energy level will be steady, and you will avoid those dangerous midday slumps that can lead to overeating.

Eating at regular intervals heals the metabolism because the body knows that energy is going to be replenished at fixed intervals. When the body knows it's in for long periods of starvation, the metabolism shuts down into "conservation mode." But with regular energy intake, the body feels secure enough to use up what it needs.

Healing the metabolism isn't about weight loss or weight gain; it's about honoring the body as an incredibly complex, incredibly beautiful organism.

6. PLAN ONE MEAL A DAY

Start off by planning the hardest meal of the day. The meal after a workout is a good beginning. Ordinarily after a workout you're so famished, you just grab whatever is convenient, like a high-fat, fast-food option. Instead of submitting to what may be a less healthful choice, try thinking through what you'll eat for that meal in advance. The positive steps you've taken by working out should help you stick to your plan. Your post-workout meal doesn't have to be elaborate—it can even be something cold such as a sandwich. Convenient fast-food fare includes fajitas, grilled or roast chicken, turkey or plain hamburger sandwiches, as well as veggie-stuffed spuds or a small order of chili. For the meal following a workout earlier in the day, you may care for something less substantial: Try half a sandwich or half a baked potato topped with grated cheese. And remember, leftovers can always work well too. Giving yourself that planned meal, nutritionally sound and thought out in advance, is a gift you'll never regret. And drinking plenty of water with each meal, especially following your workout, is yet another gift to your body.

7. CREATE CEREMONY WITH FOOD

Put effort into your food, so that what you eat nurtures you. If you want ice cream, then enjoy it, but prepare it so that it becomes a treat, something festive. Don't eat it out of the carton. Put a small scoop or two in a pretty glass and garnish with fruit; eat slowly with a long spoon. You will feel as though you've given yourself something special, and a smaller amount will satisfy.

Breakfast is another meal that can become a satisfying ceremony. When you wake up, your breakfast can be your first pleasant morning ritual. Eat your breakfast in a sunny nook, and as you enjoy coffee, cereal, milk, and fruit, contemplate this gratifying beginning of a promising and productive day.

8. DON'T SKIP BREAKFAST

Although we're largely a well-nourished country, most people overlook breakfast. I encourage clients to eat protein, complex carbohydrates, and fruit before 10:00 A.M. because the total meal gives you adequate energy after a night's fast, while the protein component provides for added satiety. Plus, breakfast can provide its share of many key nutrients, such as calcium, vitamins C and D, and folic acid. Many people say that they don't have time for breakfast. If your life is too hectic to prepare your morning meal, you may wish to simplify breakfast one or two days to a glass of milk and a piece of fruit. Even this small meal will set the stage for a more energetic and productive day.

The typical American breakfast consists of low-fat milk with breakfast cereal. But many people wonder why they're hungry so soon afterward. That's because cereal doesn't really comprise an entire meal; a little fat and protein, in the form of low-fat cheese or yogurt, or eggs, helps round it out and keeps you feeling full until snack or lunchtime. It may also help set the stage to prevent binges later on in the evening.

9. IDENTIFYING THE BINGE

Binge eating amounts to seeking nourishment where it cannot be found. If you have an urge to eat but you're not sure why, it's important to identify the feeling you're having at that time. There are numerous types of binges; for instance:

✦ The Car Binge, when you're on a long drive and wish you had some company.

✦ The Tuesday Night Binge, when it's not your night to exercise and you're eating because you don't know what else to do.

✦ The Feeling Bad Binge, when you really just need a good cry or to reach out to someone.

✦ The Anger Binge, when someone or something has annoyed or frustrated you and you're trying to dampen down your feelings of anger.

The answer to bingeing is about attending to the feelings behind it. It's also about planning meals and snacks, reinstating your relationship with yourself and your body through movement, and feeding yourself mindfully throughout the day, every day.

10. BATTLE THE BINGE

These suggestions answer the question: What else can I do? The following are self-soothing techniques that are nondestructive:

✦ Call or visit a friend
✦ Light incense or a scented candle
✦ Organize your closet
✦ Polish your nails
✦ Read a book
✦ Take a bath or shower
✦ Take a walk
✦ Tend to a pet
✦ Write down your feelings

11. IDENTIFY FOOD OPTIONS

Make a note of convenience stores near your work or home that sell fresh fruit. Or if your energy lags during the day, run to the deli for a box of raisins or yogurt instead of a candy bar. Being aware of healthier food choices at all times can help you make the best possible decisions.

For most of us food is incredibly intimate and symbolic, and it may seem daunting to attempt to change habits that have accrued over time. But if you start slowly, attempting to introduce one or two of my suggestions at a time, it won't seem like such an overwhelming project. After all, as they say, Rome wasn't built in a day! The key principles are patience, forgiveness, and a willingness to reach for long-term goals as opposed to quick fixes.

Making healthful food choices will assist in the process of self-care. It will provide your body with the fuel it needs to maintain an active routine. As with exercise, healthful eating becomes a habit, that, once achieved, continues to build a strong foundation for a lifestyle of success.

CONCLUSION

If we go down into ourselves,
we find that we possess exactly what we desire.
—Simone Weil

Now you have the tools and the program to get fit. It's all within your grasp. All the courage, all the strength, all the discipline, and all the determination already exist within you. It's just been buried—buried by a society beset with a relentless focus on thinness, which twists our thinking about ourselves; buried under layers of self-loathing; buried by the expectations of families who believe they know who we "should" be better than we do. Trust me, I know those feelings well. And while the excavation of our true selves can be overwhelming, the process is also incredibly rewarding.

Rather than trying to persuade you to conform to an unrealistic gym situation or buy into outlandish and unhealthy beauty standards, this is a program designed to help real women incorporate fitness into their lives today. Up until now you've been faced with unrealistic goals, and have been expected to come out looking like a Hollywood clone. Instead, the program outlined in *Real Fitness for Real Women* is achievable. Today. If you follow these simple suggestions, I guarantee it will change your life.

Passion is key: As a child you were probably passionate about certain physical activities, sports, dancing, and other physical games. The sheer joy of being able to feel the sun beaming down on your face or taking a walk to a friend's house filled you with glee. These simple pleasures can be yours once again. Remember your bliss, your passion. And allow that remembrance to fuel your active lifestyle, without limitations.

Creating the *Real Fitness for Real Women* program stems from my core conviction that my life's work is to help heal women and bring them back to themselves. I know instinctively that this is the work God has meant for me to do; I have never been so sure of anything in my life. At times it hasn't been easy. There have been moments when I considered returning to my former life: teaching at an unsupportive gym, eating pints of New York Super Fudge Chunk until I couldn't move, revisiting those self-hating messages. But when I recall the misery under which I used to operate, I recommit to keep moving forward. And as painful as that can be at times, it brings much more gratification than the sound of my spoon hitting the cardboard on the bottom of the ice cream container.

My life has changed so much since I began to envision different possibilities for myself and for others. It has taken years of hard work to get here, but the journey was well worth the reward. And it could not have been possible without the women I've met through my work—their faith and honesty, and their trust in me, in themselves, and in the development of this program. Now it's my turn to give back. So, dear reader, know this: You have my respect, admiration, and complete faith in your ability to accomplish this program and enjoy an active lifestyle! May this book shed some light on your journey and help guide your way.

STORIES OF INSPIRATION

I didn't belong as a kid, and that always bothered me.
If only I'd known that one day my differences would be an asset.
—Bette Midler

CYNTHIA

When thirty-two-year-old Cynthia first moved from a small town in Virginia to New York City, she found that her busy life left little time for fitness. As her level of fitness declined, she developed hypertension and was compelled to start taking medication. But today she is medication-free, managing her high blood pressure solely through diet and exercise.

I grew up in Virginia, in a little town called Amherst, where the pace of life is a lot slower, and everyone knows everyone else. I lived with my two sisters and one brother, all younger, and my mom, who worked in the social services area with foster kids and was a single parent. As the oldest child I had to take a lot of responsibility for my siblings—getting the other kids ready for school, making sure they were fed, and so on. I stayed home a lot and didn't have the same kind of social calendar that a lot of teens have.

Ours was a typical Southern house with lots of food and lots of emphasis on eating. I always loved the regional dishes, such as fried chicken, potato salad, and baked ham. My mom would prepare dishes in advance, so we could just go to the fridge and help ourselves. Most of my family is very skinny, but unfortunately I did not get those genes. I'd eat the same things they would in the same amounts they would, but they wouldn't put on weight, while it was very easy for me to get big. I felt like I didn't have any control over my weight. And no one understood. Once, my mom took me to a weight center, but since there was no support for the program at home, in the end, it didn't help. At times, family members would be very critical and tell me not to eat so much, but knocking someone down doesn't help. I just got angry at them and ate anyway.

I was a heavy teen from seventh to twelfth grade. Then all of a sudden I got very fit. I became very conscious of what I ate, and started exercising a lot. I walked and rode my bike every day, and ended up losing a good amount of weight. Then I moved to New York, and I became sedentary once again. I was working with runaway teens at Covenant House, and all of my energies were going into work. I felt like I didn't have time for fitness. I would come home exhausted and grab something quick for dinner, then collapse on the sofa. I didn't pay much attention to what I was eating. It was a mind-set thing: I just wasn't ready.

Sometimes I would try to exercise. I'd go for walks. I bought Roller Blades—they are still brand-new in my closet! I'd work out a couple days in a row and then get bored. I was trying to get my old self back, but it wasn't working. I just didn't have that drive.

Finally, a year and a half ago, I began the program in *Real Fitness for Real Women* and from the very first day began to feel more comfortable with myself. I now work out to feel better—not to lose weight, but to get fit and move. Two years ago, I was diagnosed with high blood pressure and began taking medication to control it. Now I regulate my condition through diet and exercise. I no longer need the medication. I generally work out at least once a week, but I'm building up to twice a week.

Real Fitness for Real Women has added immeasurably to my life. Currently I teach preschool and kindergarten and I have a lot more energy for the kids. I'm more active, and my daily activities are a lot easier. I don't mind doing errands, and I'm riding my bike a lot more these days. People I haven't seen for a while notice that I've lost weight, and they say I seem happier. They're right—I am!

LESLIE

Leslie battled with depression before arriving at In Fitness & In Health. At thirty, Leslie has a new lease on life. A children's therapist with a family services agency, Leslie says her workouts are the highlight of her week—energizing and empowering.

I grew up in Brooklyn with my mom, dad, and grandmother. My brother and I were heavy as children, and my grandmother used to call us "two tons." I think she thought she was doing us a favor by trying to encourage us to lose weight, but really her insults stung.

My mother, a nurse, was also very anxious about my weight, which I started gaining around age seven. She started putting me on diets when I was only eight years old. At that time, I was 32 pounds overweight, so every Saturday she would drag me to a pediatrician who put me on a special eating program. The diet didn't work, however, because my dad was secretly giving me food. He thought I was too young to be dieting, and he didn't want me to be unhappy. If I wanted a cookie or chips he'd sneak them to me. The doctor couldn't figure out why the diet wasn't working, and at first thought there was something wrong with me. She did some blood work to see if it was a thyroid condition, but finally she figured out what was going on.

When I was eleven they sent me to Weight Watchers camp. It was my first time away from home and I was very active and played a lot of sports. When I came home, I tried to continue with Weight Watchers, but I still asked my dad for junk food and he gave it to me. I put the weight back on, plus more.

My mom wasn't the only one pressuring me to lose weight—my grandmother was merciless. She would call me names, and constantly poke and pinch me. Oddly enough, she was a big woman herself. I guess she thought her tactics would keep me from being big like her.

Around eighth grade the kids got nasty. Most of them would make jokes and talk about me behind my back, but I did have some good friends who were supportive. Toward the end of high school, I started bingeing and becoming depressed. I couldn't explain what was happening, but I knew there was something wrong. I was eating a lot at night. Food began to occupy my thoughts. I would always eat, eat, eat, and tell myself I'd start a diet on Monday.

In college, I was on diet after diet. I went on a liquid diet and lost 42 pounds. But after that diet, I ate and ate, and put all the weight back on. I joined Jenny Craig for three months but couldn't stick to the eating plan. My weight went up and down, up and down. Every time I finished a dieting cycle I gained back more weight than before. By the time I was done I had put on 100 pounds.

In grad school, I made no friends, which is unusual for me. When I wasn't in class, I'd just watch TV and eat. One week all the foods I'd eat would be low-fat, and the next week I'd binge on fattening foods. Normalizing my eating habits was a constant battle.

After school I moved back home and took a job I hated. I became clinically depressed, but I didn't know it. My mom worked at a medical school nursing program at the time, and she asked the staff psychologist to see me. I was referred to a program that included counseling and antidepressants, which eventually helped the depression.

But I was still overeating and heavier than ever before. Then I learned about Rochelle's program. I enrolled in the introductory class in April of 1998 and have been going ever since. The six-week course—the program included in *Real Fitness for Real Women*—was wonderful. Even though it's just once a week, I've never been able to move like that before. I used to join gyms where I'd last a week and then quit. This time, I can't imagine quitting. I feel so much better. I like the fact that I can move and exercise and take the entire class without stopping in the middle because I feel like I am going to collapse. I used to dread the prospect of working out. Now my workout is the high point of my week. I schedule my life around my workout!

The program has made me feel like I deserve to be in the world even though I'm fat—it's okay to use the word "fat"! I no longer feel I have to wait until I'm thin to do anything. I feel empowered.

PAT

At thirty, Pat is a strikingly beautiful young woman with light brown hair, vivid green eyes, and a tall, powerful body. But her strong physical presence sharply contrasts with how she used to feel as a heavy teen—timid and shy, never dreaming that one day she'd be a fitness trainer herself.

One of my goals as a fitness trainer is eventually to work with overweight kids, because I too was overweight as a child, and I know how brutal it is to be young and not fit in. I suffered so much in my elementary school years because the other kids were incredibly cruel. They used to tease and taunt me mercilessly. At age eight, I weighed 165 pounds.

At age eleven, I weighed 200 pounds, and by the time I was thirteen, I was nearly 250 pounds at five foot ten. I knew I was fat and I felt ugly. I felt as though I was an outcast and my life wasn't worth living. Kids would pick fights with me just because they knew I wouldn't fight back. Their cruelty was so intense that I frequently stayed out of school. My mom and dad were very supportive and loving, but they just didn't know how to help me with it.

Mainly because of my poor eating habits, I developed gallstones. All the potato chips and other greasy foods I'd been eating had taken their toll on my system. It was clear I needed surgery, but the doctors didn't want to operate on me because I was so heavy. The pain became so unbearable that they finally agreed to do the surgery, but it was a difficult and embarrassing ordeal for a thirteen-year-old.

After the surgery, I stopped going to school to study at home with a tutor. Home study was great for someone like me who was exposed to so much hostility at school, but it was hardly a permanent solution. My dad and I went on Weight Watchers together and I lost 50 pounds, but eventually I started going to school again and gained it all back. I knew at the time I wasn't losing weight for myself, but to please everyone else. I tried a lot of crash diets, over-the-counter medications, and meal substitutes. The results were always short-lived.

When I graduated from high school my weight was nearing the 350 mark and I experienced a lot of job discrimination. Depression took over my life. I hated the world and myself. I got a job doing photo processing because I could just sit in the back and didn't have to deal with people. I had such low self-esteem and spent most of my time crying at home.

The turning point came in 1992 when my brother announced he was getting married. I realized that I had a year to get my weight down sufficiently so that I could wear the bridesmaid's dress without feeling awful. Something in my brain clicked. I wanted to lose weight for *me*, not because a doctor or anyone else was telling me to. This time I wanted to get fit for me.

I started changing my food habits sensibly. I began paying attention to nutrition labels, watching my fat intake, and eating salads once a day. They were satisfying meals and I'd eat all I wanted, and I wouldn't want seconds, thirds, or fourths. Instead of two hamburgers, I'd have one. By the next month, I had lost ten pounds.

I wasn't keen on self-denial, so if I wanted treats I'd allow myself to eat them in moderation. I really love candy corn, and I can eat cups and cups of it. Now I just eat a small amount and really savor it. This strategy worked very well for me; I wasn't dieting, just eating sensibly.

I started watching the exercise shows on TV and working out in the basement. I did sit-ups, crunches, and weight training. There was a lot I couldn't do at first because I was so out of shape. My dad had a NordicTrack in the house, but in the beginning my legs were too thick to use it. I couldn't last more than five minutes on the stationary bicycle. But gradually, I worked my way up. The more fit I became, the more I worked out; the more I worked out, the more energy I had. I started to feel really great, which spurred me on.

I tried to join a gym, but the trainers were very hostile. They gave me a fitness test and asked me to run up and down stairs for five minutes so they could monitor my heart rate. After two minutes, I was already out of breath. They just sat there laughing at me and rolling their eyes. The hostility didn't only come from the trainers, either. When I went into the weight room, people would stare at me or look at me like I didn't belong. I never went back. Instead I worked out at home, where it was safe and emotionally pain-free.

I kept going in for fittings of the dress and the seamstress kept having to take it in. I started out at just over 355 pounds with a 70-inch hip and a 60-inch waist. By the time the wedding arrived, I had lost 115 pounds. Soon after, there was a second wedding in our family, and by then I had lost another 50 pounds. The strangest thing happened: No one recognized me. Not even my cousins.

I realized I wanted to go into fitness professionally, start really living it. I took the American Council on Exercise personal trainer certification exam, and I began working at In Fitness & In Health in November of 1997. My life is immeasurably different from how it was before I began working out. I have a lot of great people in my life, a lot of friends. I am living and enjoying my life to the fullest.

KATHLEEN

Kathleen is no stranger to life's ups and downs. The 1990s were a tough decade for her, during which she experienced the death of both parents as well as a divorce. But this thirty-six-year-old legal secretary is a true survivor.

I grew up in a working-class home in New Jersey with my sister and two brothers. My mom spent her days working in a small accounting firm, and my dad worked all sorts of hours as a railroad engineer. Our life as a family was organized around dinnertime. Sitting around the table every night was where we got back in touch with each other, and no excuses were accepted for missing this daily ritual.

We are a family of full-sized people. My dad was a big guy, tall and heavyset. My mom was a beautiful redhead, teetering on the edge of plus size. Though I was fairly active as a kid, there really wasn't a lot of emphasis put on exercise. In school, I was a little different from the other kids because I was big, but it never really stood in my way. I was president of my senior class, went to a lot of dances, and dated plenty of guys. When I was fifteen years old, I met the boy whom, ten years later, I would marry.

When I was twenty-eight both of my parents died of unrelated illnesses. It was a traumatic year, during which I started taking less care of myself. I wasn't concerned with my own well-being.

Five years after that my husband and I got divorced. I felt betrayed, and a little afraid. I began to lose my femininity, my attractiveness, and my worthiness as a woman. I felt very insecure.

At first I was too busy trying to keep it all together to take care of myself, but after a while I wanted to do something physical—something that would put me back in charge. I joined In Fitness & In Health and began Rochelle's exercise program.

Working out helped me to get back my physical and emotional strength. It was an incredibly empowering experience. At first I was terrified I would try it and not stick to it, but with Rochelle that was not a problem. At the end of six weeks I felt better. I began to look forward to the challenge and the discipline.

Working out has made me more aware of my own body and the kindnesses that I can show to myself. It's a lot easier for me to make better food choices as well. I haven't been dieting, I've just become more aware of what I'm eating. These small changes make such a big difference in the quality of life. It's taken me every moment of my thirty-six years to figure that out.

I feel confident now when I walk in the street. And at the end of my workouts, instead of feeling completely exhausted, I feel elated.

BARBARA

Barbara, fifty-six, is a nurse practitioner, psychotherapist, and author who began using the program in Real Fitness for Real Women *in 1998. Her company encourages women who are in the nursing profession to empower themselves. She is a consultant at a number of hospitals, is a mental health clinician for Lenox Hill Hospital, and teaches at NYU and Mercy College. Her struggle with her size has led her to some incisive conclusions about society's prejudices toward large women.*

When I was growing up in the 1950s, there was very little awareness of fitness, especially for girls. It wasn't acceptable for girls to play sports, and there were no fitness salons—only boxing gyms. I had gym class at school but I hated it, and nobody encouraged me to be physical. Around that time, though,

President Kennedy made physical fitness a national goal. From then on people started to think about fitness in a different way.

I was an overweight child beginning from age eight or nine. Like all kids I wanted to fit in with my peers, so being big wounded my self-esteem. My family ignored my weight problem. I felt as though there was a certain denial about it. They would say I was really beautiful and shouldn't worry about what people thought of me. But it felt as though they just weren't acknowledging the extent of my problem.

We are an Italian-American family, and dinners were always large. My grandmother and mother were both overweight, and during the holidays they literally spent days preparing the food. A dinner might last from early afternoon until the middle of the evening. We always had some kind of appetizer like an antipasto, tons of bread, soup, a roast, all the vegetables and trimmings. Then the pasta would come, pastries that lasted forever, then nuts. Every holiday was centered around the dining table.

After high school I went to nursing school in Brooklyn, and went from there into the Army Nurse Corps. When I left four years later, the military was starting to make physical fitness more of a focus, even for the doctors and nurses. That certainly wasn't the reason I left, but it was one factor.

I was still overweight and not happy about it, so eventually in the 1970s I started to go to the gym. However, like a lot of plus-size women, I did not find the gym to be a welcoming place. In order for a large woman to be able to go to a traditional gym, she has to do so much work on herself internally, deciding she isn't going to pay attention to how people view her. It's an enormous undertaking—to wall off what you know is going on in other people's heads. It takes up so much energy and left me depressed. Like many large people, I tend to internalize the negative messages about large women I get from the culture, and that's almost impossible to fight. In addition I have to fight the battle everyone has to fight—motivating myself to work out. So there are always two battles going on, which makes it that much harder to get myself to work out.

I've gotten thin five times, but my experience is that it's hard to maintain. I'd succeed in getting my weight down, but like a boomerang, it would bounce back up immediately. I tried Optifast, I joined Weight Watchers many times, and earlier in my life I tried diet drugs and amphetamines. The weight never stayed off. So five years ago I decided to try something different. I lost about 60 pounds and this time I stopped myself on purpose because I wanted to practice maintaining that weight loss. In five years I've put back only 20 of those pounds, and that's a big success for me.

I discovered In Fitness & In Health and the program in *Real Fitness for Real Women* through a friend. I began with one workout a week. It was hard in the beginning, but I now work out about three times a week.

I never thought I would enjoy the experience of getting fit. Now I have a different attitude about myself and my body. I think, "If you don't like the way I look, then look someplace else!" I am experiencing a freedom, not just intellectually, but throughout my spirit. I feel much more willing to let my inner strength carry me through.

You can't disconnect the physical and the spiritual. The program in *Real Fitness for Real Women* helps connect them. I'm beginning to be aware of my connection to my muscles and my body, as well as to my spirit. I have more stamina, mental clarity, and energy. I feel more alive!

DENYSE

Fifty-seven-year-old Denyse has lived in Manhattan all her life. After thirty-two years working for the same bank, she took early retirement. And that's when her troubles began. She became more sedentary and experienced a post-retirement depression, but the program in Real Fitness for Real Women *has helped her cope.*

My two sisters and I grew up with my grandmother and my mother. Many of my family members were heavy. My grandmother was heavy. She was my height—about five one—and always weighed over 200 pounds. My mother wasn't fat, but she was "built." I was always the shortest and smallest. I never played sports because it was the 1940s and 1950s and girls just didn't. As a child, I never gave mealtime any thought because I was such a picky eater. My grandma had to invent tricks to get me to eat.

In my twenties and thirties I used to go to exercise classes regularly. It was during the 1980s that things started getting so busy on the job that I fell out of the habit. When I retired, I tried to become active again. Three times a week I would walk around the neighborhood. During that time I slimmed down a bit. But when winter set in, my real problems began. I had never been one to suffer from winter depression, but with no work for the first time in my life, I was going nuts. That's when the weight started to pile on. I would sit in my house, and if it looked dreary I wouldn't go out.

Occasionally a friend and I would take a stretch and tone class at the local high school, but when winter set in again, I would sit in my favorite spot on the couch and crochet, munching potato chips.

I started getting mad at myself for not doing anything. I can always tell when I start putting on weight because I become short of breath when I walk. So finally, sometime last year, I was fed up with feeling bad about myself and said, "Okay, I'm really going to do it this time."

It was rough getting into it at first. I had a bad habit of starting exercise classes and quitting after a few weeks. But this time I kept it up. I began working out at In Fitness & In Health and doing the program in *Real Fitness for Real Women*, and so far it's been good. It's very rewarding, though you need a lot of patience. Since I also teach an adult literacy class, I can only fit two workouts a week into my schedule.

I find myself walking better now and I'm not winded all the time. Before I started this program, when I'd walk around the neighborhood I'd have to walk slowly and take breaks now and then. Now I can walk without any problems.

My best friend supports me a lot. She'll say, "Oh Denyse, you look different. Are you losing weight?" I'll say, "No, it's just shifting!" I went to my doctor and I haven't lost weight, but my clothes fit a lot better, so I know my shape is changing. I can tell when I put on my slacks. I notice I have a shape—no bulges anymore. My eating habits haven't changed much. I was on a healthy eating regimen from a nutritionist, and I try to maintain the habit, but I slip now and then. I'm still a potato chip junkie! But I do eat more fruit, drink more juice and water since I started working out, and that's an improvement. Since I started this program I feel more energetic. I don't get depressed the way I used to, and I no longer feel annoyed with myself for not being in shape.

ANITA

Anita, thirty-eight, is a lecturer, education administrator, and former director of a Head Start program. She has a husband and two children. After two difficult pregnancies that compelled her to become sedentary, she is active once again.

Both my parents are from the South, where there's a tradition of heavy cooking. In our family almost everybody is overweight to some degree, so being big is not looked at as anything strange, that's just how you are. When I stopped eating such heavy food, some members of my family got upset. When I declined dishes such as fried chicken or pork, I got the feeling they were saying to themselves, "How come you don't eat that way now? Do you think you're better than us?" In families, food can be very emotional.

Once I got to college I became very active. I started running daily, partied a lot, and slimmed down. My problems with weight began with my first pregnancy. When it came time to give birth I was in labor from Saturday until Monday. My son weighed eight pounds, eight ounces, and he just wouldn't come out! Finally we had to do a C-section.

That experience set me back in terms of fitness. A cesarean is much harder on the body than a normal birth—you have all the recuperation processes of surgery. In addition to all the stresses of a new baby, I had to deal with pressures from work. I had just received my first promotion to an administrative job and had to be back in the office in eight weeks.

After that first pregnancy I went to Weight Watchers and lost a lot of weight. But after I slimmed down I got pregnant again. I did not expect to have another C-section, but after twenty hours in labor with my daughter, I had to have another one.

This time I was prepared emotionally, but a few days later the stitches opened. So they used staples on my stomach, which hurt like crazy! I had to be very careful, which meant I stayed away from exercise for about a year. And the weight I had gained with my son all came back, and then some.

Since I've joined In Fitness & In Health and have been following the program in *Real Fitness for Real Women*, the shape of my body has changed. I now have contours again. When people tell you you're looking better you know it's worth it. I had tried other gyms, but I got tired of people saying, "You know, for someone of your size you do really well." I needed to be unconcerned with my size and just do what I do. I now feel more connected with my body than before; I'm learning to breathe correctly, and that enables me to move correctly and strengthen my abdomen again.

My husband has been supportive of me throughout everything, including both of my pregnancies. He is from Panama and used to be a swimmer, and now he works out to avoid having problems with his back. Sometimes I exercise with my kids as well, so it's something the whole family does.

Last month my little cousin Jennifer started working out with me. She's twelve, a big girl, five eight, a little overweight, and I talked to her about working out because she's at an age where she can get self-conscious about her body. She has been my workout partner for two months. I'm in her life to help shape those pre-teenage years, and this is one of the positive things I can do. Now she'll call me and say, "Are we going to work out today?" She is naturally athletic and loves strength training. Other girls her age don't work with weights yet, so this gives her an advantage.

Large women are the majority of America. Walk down the street and look at people, and you'll see. Most gyms target people who are thin or small. So it's good to have a workout program tailored to me, rather than trying to fit into somebody else's idea of fitness.

SANDY

Sandy, forty-three, was a large child, and she was endlessly hounded about her weight by her family—which only made the problem worse. Today she has two life passions: political activism and fitness. Sandy is living proof that a woman can be physically fit and plus size.

My mother has always told me that I was the only baby to gain weight before leaving the hospital. At three months, on a doctor's advice, she put me on my first of many diets.

For as long as I can remember, my weight was an overwhelming issue in my life. My parents watched me constantly to see what I was eating and treated my weight as a sign of moral weakness. When I was ten, my doctor told my mother that I would be heavy all my life because that's the way I was built. My mother couldn't accept that. Instead, my parents bribed and cajoled me into trying every diet under the sun. By the time I was twelve years old I had tried a low-carbohydrate, all-protein diet; a yogurt diet; a banana diet; a milk shake diet; a fasting, no-food diet; Weight Watchers; and a three-items-a-day revolving-food-plan diet—to name a few. None of them worked. I often wondered where I'd gone wrong.

Though I had friends and was involved in drama in high school, I never really felt a part of school life. High school gym class was a lesson in humiliation. I stayed away from any activities in which attention would be called to my weight.

After college I led a life that was active and meaningful. I walked, swam at the beach, went through a period during which I took tai chi training. Several times, I tried joining gyms, but I felt intimidated and uncomfortable.

Despite these setbacks, it wasn't until I started at the job I have now, working at a musician's union, that I became more sedentary and got really out of shape. I was huffing and puffing after walking a few blocks. Climbing the stairs to my fifth-floor apartment, my heart would pound hard and I'd lose my breath. I was afraid I would have a heart attack. I felt more and more isolated and alienated from life. I saw the future: One day I wouldn't be able to walk out of my apartment.

Frightened, I decided that I had to do something. I thought that I needed to lose weight. I went to a diet doctor who said, "If any diet is going to work, you've got to exercise as well."

First I joined a gym near work and took what they called a low-impact aerobics class. There were no other heavy people in the room. The pace was very fast and it was a struggle to keep up as the instructor shouted "Knees up, Knees up" over the loud music. They had us doing jumping jacks, a high-impact move. There was no instruction in technique. I would try imitating other people stretching, because I didn't know how or what to stretch. I wished there was a class on how to exercise, but there was none.

I noticed that I wasn't the only heavy person at the gym, but I was the only one taking classes. All the other people of size would either work out on their own on the bicycle or treadmill, or swim. I soon followed suit. Although I had paid as much money as everyone else, it just didn't feel like my place. I described this problem to a friend of mine at a party. She told me she was going to an exercise studio called In Fitness & In Health that catered to heavy women.

From the very first workout I felt at home. I began on the six-week program in *Real Fitness for Real Women*. I felt challenged, not out of my league. Soon I was working out three or four times a week. I was hooked.

This program has reconnected me with my body—a body I'd spent my life running away from. Before long, I was able to move more easily. I won't say that I started running up my stairs, but my breathing improved immediately and I started feeling good. In a few months, my whole shape changed dramatically.

I was still seeing the diet doctor, but after a time, I stopped losing weight. When I asked him about it, he said, "Are you kidding? You're my success story! You've increased your activities, you've lowered your cholesterol and blood pressure, and you have a much more upbeat outlook on life."

Since the day I dove in with both sneakers, everything has changed. Becoming fit and in tune with my body saved my life and has made me feel more part of the world, more entitled to all that it has to offer. I have become more aggressive at work and more willing to take risks.

I had been working out at In Fitness & In Health for almost two years when I began teaching exercise. I finally decided to become an instructor because exercise had become my passion. I stopped listening to the message that thin was better, and when I no longer allowed that message to make me feel excluded and unentitled, I changed my own perception of myself. In turn, the world's perception of me changed as well—or maybe it just stopped being important.

RESOURCES

While there are many resources available, I have listed a few of my favorites to help get you started on your journey.

FITNESS WEAR AND PRODUCTS

Amplestuff: PO Box 116, Bearsville, NY 12409; (845) 679-3316; www.amplestuff.com.

Champion Sportswear: 5 New England Drive, Essex Junction, VT 05452; www.championjogbra.com.

Danskin Plus: (800) 288-6749 or visit On Stage, 197 Madison Avenue, New York, NY 10016 or Danskin at 159 Columbus Avenue, New York, NY 10023.

In Fitness & In Health: 200 East 35th Street, Suite 2, New York, NY 10016; (877) 943-7749 or (212) 689-4558; www.infitnessinhealth.com.

Junonia: 800 Transfer Road, Suite 8, St. Paul, MN 55114; (800) 671-0175; www.junonia.com.

Just My Size: (800) 522-9567 or (888) 567-3487; www.justmysize.net.

Plus Woman: 85 Laurel Haven, Fairview, NC 28730; (800) 628-5525; www.pluswoman.com.

ORGANIZATIONS

The American Anorexia Bulimia Association, Inc. (AABA): AABA is a national nonprofit organization dedicated to the prevention, treatment, and cure of eating disorders. 165 West 46th Street, Suite 1108, New York, NY 10036; (212) 575-6200; www.aabainc.org.

Council on Size & Weight Discrimination, Inc.: The Council is committed to their mission, which is to influence public opinion and policy in order to end discrimination based on body size, shape, or weight. They work to make the world a safer place for people who are larger than average. PO Box 305, Mount Marion, NY 12456; (845) 679-1209; www.cswd.org.

Eating Disorders Awareness and Prevention (EDAP): EDAP is dedicated to education about and prevention of eating disorders. They also organize an annual Eating Disorders Awareness Week each February. 603 Stewart Street, Suite 803, Seattle, WA 98101; (206) 292-9890; http://members.aol.com/edapinc.

Largesse—Resource Network for Size Esteem: P.O. Box 9404, New Haven, CT 06534-0404; (203) 787-1624; www.largesse.com.

The National Association to Advance Fat Acceptance (NAAFA): NAAFA is a nonprofit human rights organization dedicated to improving the quality of life for people of size. PO Box 188620, Sacramento, CA 95818; (916) 558-6880; www.naafa.org.

BOOKS

Berg, Frances M., *Women Afraid to Eat: Breaking Free in Today's Weight-Obsessed World* (Healthy Weight Network, 2000).

Brandan, Nathaniel, *How to Raise Your Self-Esteem* (Bantam Books, 1987).

Erdman, Cheri, *Nothing to Lose* (Harper San Francisco, 1995).

Ernsberger, Paul, and Paul Haskew, "Re-thinking Obesity: An Alternative View of Its Health Implications," in *Journal of Obesity and Weight Regulation*,1987.

Fraser, Laura, *Losing It: False Hopes and Fat Profits in the Diet Industry* (Plume, 1998).

Gaesser, Glenn, *Big Fat Lies* (Fawcett Columbine, 1996).

Goodman, Charisse, *The Invisible Woman: Confronting Weight Prejudice in America* (Gurze Books, 1995).

Hays, Kate F., *Working It Out: Using Exercise in Psychotherapy* (American Psychological Association, 1999).

Hirschman, Jane, and Carol Munter, *Overcoming Overeating* (Fawcett Columbine, 1988).

———, *When Women Stop Hating Their Bodies* (Ballantine, 1995).

Johnson, Carol, *Self-Esteem Comes in All Sizes: How to Be Healthy and Happy at Your Natural Weight* (Doubleday, 1995).

Johnson, Karen, *Trusting Ourselves: The Complete Guide to Emotional Well-Being for Women* (Atlantic Monthly Press, 1991).

Lyons, Pat, and Debora Burgard, *Great Shape: The First Fitness Guide for Large Women* (Bull Publishing, 1988).

Maine, Margo, *Body Wars: Making Peace with Women's Bodies* (Gurze Books, 2000).

Northrup, Christine, *Women's Bodies, Women's Wisdom: Creating Physical and Emotional Health and Healing* (Bantam, 1994).

Sullivan, Judy, *Size Wise: A Catalog of More Than 1000 Resources for Living Large with Confidence and Comfort at Any Size* (Avon Books, 1997).

MAGAZINES AND JOURNALS

BBW: Big Beautiful Women: Aeon Publishing Co., 4045 Sunset Lane, Suite A, Shingle Springs, CA 95682; (877) BBW-STYLE; www.bbwmagazine.com.

Belle: 474 Park Avenue South, New York, NY 10016; (800) 877-5549 or (212) 689-2830.

Fat!So?: PO Box 423464, San Francisco, CA 94142-3464.

Healthy Weight Journal: Healthy Living Institute, 402 South 14th Street, Hettinger, ND 58639; (701) 567-2646.

Largely Positive Newsletter: Carol Johnson, Director, PO Box 17223, Glendale, WI 53217-8021; (414) 299-9295; Positive@execpc.com.

MODE: 1040 Sixth Avenue, New York, NY 10018; (888) 610-MODE; www.modemag.com.

Radiance: The Magazine for Large Women: PO Box 30246, Oakland, CA 94604; (510) 482-0680; www.radiancemagazine.com.

WEB SITES

Grandstyle.com: fashion, fitness, and fun for sizes 14 and up.

Health at Any Size: www.bodypositive.com.

Plus Stop: www.plusstop.com.

Thrive: www.thriveonline.com.

INDEX